# TABLE OF CONTENTS

*Copyright © Mometrix Media. You have been licensed one copy of this document for personal use only.*
*Any other reproduction or redistribution is strictly prohibited. All rights reserved.*

*Copyright © Mometrix Media. You have been licensed one copy of this document for personal use only.*
*Any other reproduction or redistribution is strictly prohibited. All rights reserved.*

# Top 20 Test Taking Tips

1. Carefully follow all the test registration procedures
2. Know the test directions, duration, topics, question types, how many questions
3. Setup a flexible study schedule at least 3-4 weeks before test day
4. Study during the time of day you are most alert, relaxed, and stress free
5. Maximize your learning style; visual learner use visual study aids, auditory learner use auditory study aids
6. Focus on your weakest knowledge base
7. Find a study partner to review with and help clarify questions
8. Practice, practice, practice
9. Get a good night's sleep; don't try to cram the night before the test
10. Eat a well balanced meal
11. Know the exact physical location of the testing site; drive the route to the site prior to test day
12. Bring a set of ear plugs; the testing center could be noisy
13. Wear comfortable, loose fitting, layered clothing to the testing center; prepare for it to be either cold or hot during the test
14. Bring at least 2 current forms of ID to the testing center
15. Arrive to the test early; be prepared to wait and be patient
16. Eliminate the obviously wrong answer choices, then guess the first remaining choice
17. Pace yourself; don't rush, but keep working and move on if you get stuck
18. Maintain a positive attitude even if the test is going poorly
19. Keep your first answer unless you are positive it is wrong
20. Check your work, don't make a careless mistake

*Copyright © Mometrix Media. You have been licensed one copy of this document for personal use only. Any other reproduction or redistribution is strictly prohibited. All rights reserved.*

# Clinical Judgment
## *Cardiovascular*

**Angina**

Unstable:
Unstable angina (also known as preinfarction or crescendo angina) is a progression of coronary artery disease and occurs when there is a change in the pattern of stable angina. The pain from angina may increase, may not respond to a single nitroglycerine, and may persist for >5 minutes. Usually pain is more frequent, lasts longer, and may occur at rest. Unstable angina may indicate rupture of an atherosclerotic plaque and the beginning of thrombus formation. It should always be treated as a medical emergency as it may indicate a myocardial infarction

Variant:
Variant angina (also known as Prinzmetal's angina) results from spasms of the coronary arteries associated with or without atherosclerotic plaques and is often related to smoking, alcohol, or illicit stimulants. Elevation of ST segments usually occurs with variant angina. Variant angina frequently occurs cyclically, i.e., at the same time each day, and often while the person is at rest. Nitroglycerine or calcium channel blockers are used for treatment.

**Myocardial infarction**

Myocardial infarction (MI) occurs when there is an imbalance between the heart's demand for oxygen and the supply. An MI is part of the continuum of acute coronary syndrome (ACS) and may occur after an episode of unstable angina caused by rupture of an atherosclerotic plaque and thrombosis associated with coronary artery spasm. An MI may also result from vasoconstriction, acute blood loss, decreased oxygen, and ingestion of cocaine. Damage to the myocardium typically occurs in stages, beginning in the endocardium and progressing to the epicardium:
- Ischemia develops as oxygen levels fall, creating a *zone of ischemia* with viable cells.
- Cellular injury occurs to those cells surrounding the infarcted area in the *zone of injury.*

Infarction with necrosis of tissue occurs in the *zone of infarction,* where cells are destroyed and eventually replaced with scar tissue. Irreversible damage occurs with complete occlusion for 15 to 20 minutes.

Q-wave and non-Q-wave myocardial infarctions:
Myocardial infarctions (formerly classified as transmural or non-transmural) are currently classified as Q-wave or non-Q-wave:
***Q-wave:*** Characterized by series of abnormal Q waves (wider and deeper) on ECG, especially in the early AM (related to adrenergic activity). Infarction is usually prolonged and results in necrosis.
Coronary occlusion is complete in 80%-90%.
Q-wave MI is often, but not always, transmural.
Peak CK levels occur in about 27 hours.
Mortality rates are about 10%.

***Non-Q-wave:*** Characterized by changes in ST-T wave with ST depression (usually reversible within a few days).
Usually reperfusion occurs spontaneously, so infarct size is smaller. Contraction necrosis related to reperfusion is common.
Non-Q-wave MI is usually non-transmural.
Coronary occlusion is complete in only 20%-30%.
Peak CK levels occur in 12-13 hours.
Mortality rates are about 2%-3%.
Reinfarction is common, so 2-year survival rates are similar to Q-wave MI.

Areas of occlusion:
A myocardial infarction most frequently damages the left ventricle and the septum, but the right ventricle may be damaged, depending upon the occluded area:
- ***Anterior wall infarction*** occurs with occlusion in the proximal left anterior descending artery and may damage the left ventricle.
- ***Left lateral wall infarction*** occurs with occlusion of the circumflex coronary artery

*Copyright © Mometrix Media. You have been licensed one copy of this document for personal use only.*
*Any other reproduction or redistribution is strictly prohibited. All rights reserved.*

and often causes damage to anterior wall as well.

- **Inferior wall infarction** occurs with occlusion of the right coronary artery and causes conduction malfunctions.
- **Right ventricular infarction** occurs with occlusion of the proximal section of the right coronary artery and damages the right ventricle and the inferior wall.
- **Posterior wall infarction** occurs with occlusion in the right coronary artery or circumflex artery and may be difficult to diagnose.

Clinical manifestations:

Clinical manifestations of myocardial infarction may vary considerably, with males having the more "classic" symptom of sudden onset of crushing chest pain, in contrast to females and individuals under the age of 55 who present with atypical symptoms. Diabetic patients may have reduced sensation of pain because of neuropathy and may complain primarily of weakness. Elderly patients may also have neuropathic changes that reduce sensation of pain. More than half of all patients present with acute MIs with no prior symptoms of cardiovascular disease. Symptoms may include:

- Angina with pain in chest that may radiate to neck or arms.
- Palpitations.
- Hypertension or hypotension.
- Electrocardiogram (ECG) changes (ST segment and T-wave changes, tachycardia, bradycardia, and dysrhythmias).
- Dyspnea, pulmonary edema.
- Nausea and vomiting, indigestion.
- Decreased urinary output.
- Pallor, skin cold and clammy, diaphoresis.
- Dependent edema.
- Neurological/psychological disturbances: anxiety, light-headed, headache, visual abnormalities, slurred speech, and fear.

Diagnostic procedures:

Diagnosis of a myocardial infarction includes a complete physical examination, a patient and family history, and an assessment of risk factors. Assessment may include:

- *ECG* obtained immediately to monitor heart changes over time. Typical changes include T-wave inversion, elevation of ST segment, and abnormal Q waves.
- *Echocardiogram* to evaluate ventricular function.
- *Creatine kinase (CK) and isoenzyme (MB)*:
  o CK-MB (cardiac muscle) level increases within a few hours and peaks at about 24-27 hours (earlier with thrombolytic therapy or PTCA) for Q-wave MI and at about 12-13 hours for non-Q-wave.
- *Myoglobin* (heme protein that transports oxygen) found in both skeletal and cardiac muscles. Levels increase in 1-3 hours after an MI and peak within 12 hours. While an increase is not specific to an MI, a failure to increase can be used to rule out an MI.
- *Troponin* (protein in the myocardium) and its isomers (C, I, and T) regulate contraction and their levels increase as with CK-MB, but levels remains elevated for up to 3 weeks.

**Papillary muscle rupture**

The atrioventricular valves separate the atria from the ventricles with the tricuspid valve on the right and the bicuspid (mitral) valve on the left. The *papillary muscles* are located on the sides of ventricular walls and connect to the valves with fibrous bands called chordae tendineae. During systole, the papillary muscles contract, tightening the chordae tendineae and closing the valves. One complication of an MI is papillary muscle rupture, usually on the left affecting the mitral valve, with the posteromedial papillary muscle more often affected than the anterolateral. Dysfunction of the papillary muscles occurs in about 40% of those with a posterior-septal infarction, but rupture can occur with infarction of the inferior wall or with an anterolateral MI. Rupture on the right side results in tricuspid regurgitation and right ventricular failure, whereas rupture on the left side leads to mitral regurgitation with resultant pulmonary edema and cardiogenic

*Copyright © Mometrix Media. You have been licensed one copy of this document for personal use only. Any other reproduction or redistribution is strictly prohibited. All rights reserved.*

shock. Early identification of the papillary muscles affected and surgical repair is critical.

## Myocarditis

Myocarditis is inflammation of the cardiac myocardium (muscle tissue), usually triggered by a viral infection such as the influenza virus, Coxsackie virus, and HIV. Myocarditis can also be caused by bacteria, fungi, and parasites or by an allergic response to medications. In some cases, it is also a complication of endocarditis. It may also be triggered by chemotherapy drugs and some antibiotics. Myocarditis can result in dilation of the heart, development of thrombi on the heart walls (known as mural thrombi), and infiltration of blood cells around the coronary vessels and between muscle fibers, conditions that cause further degeneration of the muscle tissue. The heart may become enlarged and weak as the ability to pump blood is impaired, leading to congestive heart failure. *Symptoms* depend upon the extent of damage but may include fatigue, dyspnea, pressure and discomfort in chest or epigastric area, and palpitations.

Diagnosis and treatment:
Diagnosis of myocarditis depends upon the clinical picture because there is no test specific for myocarditis, although a number of tests may be done to verify the clinical diagnosis:

- Chest radiograph may indicate cardiomegaly or pulmonary edema.
- ECG may show non-specific changes.
- Echocardiogram may indicate cardiomegaly and defects in functioning.
- Cardiac catheterization and cardiac biopsy will yield confirmation in 65% of cases, but not all of the heart muscle may be affected, so a negative finding does not rule out myocarditis.
- Viral cultures of nasopharynx and rectal may help to identify organism.
- Viral titers may increase as disease progresses.
- Polymerase chain reaction (PCR) of biopsy specimen may be most effective test for diagnosis.

*Treatment*:
- As indicated to correct underlying cause (such as antibiotics).
- Restriction of activities.
- Careful monitoring for heart failure and medical treatment as indicated (diuretics, digoxin, etc.).
- Oxygen as needed to maintain normal oxygen saturation.
- IV gamma globulin for acute stage.

## Pericarditis

Pericarditis is inflammation of the pericardial membrane that surrounds the heart. The outer fibrous pericardium is connective tissue that is continuous with the outer layers of the great vessels and serves to protect and anchor the heart. The inner serous pericardium has 2 layers separated with serous pericardial fluid to lubricate the heart and prevent friction. With pericarditis, the layers may become attached to each other (dry), or the serous fluid may be replaced by purulent material, calcifications, fibrinous material, or blood. Pericarditis is frequently associated with surgical repair of cardiac structural abnormalities, but it may also result from other systemic viral, bacterial, fungal, and parasitic infections or may be caused by direct trauma. Some chronic connective tissue disorders, such as lupus erythematosus, may also cause pericarditis. Pericarditis is often accompanied by fever, dysrhythmia, poor appetite, irritability, malaise, and sharp, piercing chest pain.

Diagnosis and treatment:
Pericarditis is treated according to the cause and the type and extent of inflammation. *Diagnostic* procedures are similar to those for endocarditis and myocarditis. *Treatment* includes:
- Analgesics as indicated to control pain.
- Anti-inflammatory drugs, aspirin or ibuprofen, may be used to relieve discomfort and increase the rate of fluid reabsorption.
- Restriction of activity is necessary if cardiac function and output is impaired.

Copyright © Mometrix Media. You have been licensed one copy of this document for personal use only. Any other reproduction or redistribution is strictly prohibited. All rights reserved.

- Corticosteroids are used in some cases if there is no response to anti-inflammatory drugs.
- Surgical intervention may include pericardiocentesis, which is removing fluid from the pericardial sac in order to relieve increasing pressure and to diagnose the causative agent. In some cases, a small opening may be made into the pericardium to allow continuous drainage of exudate into the chest cavity. In severe cases, the outer layer of the pericardium may need to be removed if it is preventing functioning of the ventricles.

## Endocarditis

Endocarditis is an infection of the endothelial surface and valves of the heart. It is caused by invasion of the tissue by a pathogen, commonly streptococci, staphylococci, enterococci, pneumococci as well as fungi and rickettsia. The infection is often hospital-acquired. Organisms enter the bloodstream from portals of entry (surgery, catheterization, IV drug abuse) and migrate to the heart, growing on the endothelial tissue and forming vegetations (verrucae), collagen deposits, and platelet thrombi. With endocarditis, the valves frequently become deformed, but the pathogenic agents may also invade other tissues, such as the chordae tendineae. The lesions may invade adjacent tissue and break off, becoming emboli. Endocarditis is associated with prolonged hospitalization, recent cardiac surgery (especially with synthetic grafts or valves), presence of pulmonary shunts, invasive devices (such as central lines), congenital heart disease, as well as rheumatic heart disease with involvement of valves.

Clinical symptoms:
Clinical symptoms of endocarditis usually relate to the response to infection, the underlying heart disease, emboli, or immunological response. Typical *symptoms* include:
- Slow onset with unexplained low-grade and often intermittent fever.
- Anorexia and weight loss, difficulty feeding.

- General lassitude and malaise.
- Splenomegaly (in 60%) and hepatomegaly.
- Anemia is present in almost all patients.
- Sudden aortic valve insufficiency or mitral valve insufficiency.
- Cyanosis with clubbing of fingers.
- Embolism of other body organs (brain, liver, bones).
- Congestive heart failure.
- Dysrhythmias, new or change in heart murmur.
- Immunological responses:
  o Janeway lesions: painless areas of hemorrhage on palms of hands and soles of feet.
  o Splinter hemorrhages: thin, brown-black lines on nails of fingers and toes.
  o Petechiae on oral mucous membranes, as well as hands and trunk.
  o Roth's spots: hemorrhagic lesions on the retina caused by emboli on nerve fibers.
  o Glomerulonephritis with hematuria found on microscopy.

Diagnosis and treatment:
*Diagnosis* of endocarditis is made on the basis of clinical presentation and diagnostic procedures that may include:
- Blood cultures should be done with 3 sets for both aerobic and anaerobic bacteria. Diagnosis is definitive if 2 cultures are positive, but a negative culture does not preclude bacterial endocarditis.
- Echocardiogram may identify vegetation on valves or increasing heart failure.
- ECG may demonstrate prolonged P-R interval.
- Anemia (normochromic, normocytic).
- Elevated white cell count.
- Elevated erythrocyte sedimentation rate (ESR) and C-reactive protein (CRP).

*Treatment* includes general management of symptoms and the following:
- Antimicrobials specific to the pathogenic organism, usually administered intravenously for 4-6 weeks.

*Copyright © Mometrix Media. You have been licensed one copy of this document for personal use only. Any other reproduction or redistribution is strictly prohibited. All rights reserved.*

- Surgical replacement of aortic and/or mitral valves may be necessary (in 30%-40% of cases) if there is no response to treatment and/or after infection is controlled, if there are severe symptoms related to valve damage.

**Repairing cardiac valves**

There are a number of different surgical options for repair of cardiac valves:

- *Valvotomy/Valvuloplasty* is usually done through cardiac catheterization. A valvotomy/valvuloplasty may involve releasing valve leaflet adhesions interfering with functioning of the valve. In balloon valvuloplasty, a catheter with an inflatable balloon is positioned in the stenotic valve and inflated and deflated a number of times to dilate the opening.
- *Aortic valve replacement* is an open-heart procedure with cardiopulmonary bypass. Aortic valves are tricuspid (3 leaflets) and repair is usually not possible, so defective valves must be replaced with either mechanical (metal, plastic, or pyrolytic carbon) or biological (porcine or bovine xenografts).
- *Aortic homograft* uses part of a donor's aorta with the aortic valve attached to replace the recipient's faulty aortic valve and part of the ascending aorta.
- *Ross procedure* uses the patient's pulmonary artery with the pulmonary valve to replace the aortic valve and part of the aorta and then uses a donor graft to replace the pulmonary artery.

**Coronary artery bypass graft**

Coronary artery bypass graft (CABG) is a surgical procedure for treatment of angina that does not respond to medical treatment, unstable angina, blockage of >60% in left main coronary artery, blockage of multiple coronary arteries that include the proximal left anterior descending artery, left ventricular dysfunction, and previous unsuccessful percutaneous coronary interventions (PCIs). The surgery is performed through a midsternal incision that exposes the heart, which is chilled and placed on cardiopulmonary bypass (CPB) with blood going from the right atrium to the machine and back to the body while the aorta is clamped to keep the surgical field free of blood. Bypass grafts are sutured into place to bypass areas of occluded coronary arteries. Grafts may be obtained from various sites:

- Gastroepiploic artery.
- Internal mammary artery (commonly used and superior to saphenous vein, but procedure is more time-consuming).
- Radial artery.
- Saphenous vein (commonly used, especially for emergency procedures).

Postoperative complications include MI, graft failure, occlusion of other arteries, dysrhythmias, emboli, and infection.

**Intraaortic balloon pump**

The intraaortic balloon (IAB) pump is the most commonly used circulatory assist device. It is used for a number of problems (unstable angina, myocardial infarction, cardiogenic shock, papillary muscle dysfunction, ventricular failure after cardiac surgery, and dysrhythmias), and it may be used to facilitate weaning patients from CPB after open-heart surgery if the heart is not able to pump adequately. The IAB comprises a 90-cm stiff catheter with a 25-cm inflatable balloon from the tip and lengthwise down the catheter. The catheter is usually inserted through the femoral artery but may be placed during surgery or through a cutdown. The catheter is threaded into the descending thoracic aorta, and the balloon inflates during diastole to increase circulation to the coronary arteries and then deflates during systole to decrease afterload. Complications can include dysrhythmias, peripheral ischemia from femoral artery occlusion, and balloon perforation or migration. Tachycardia and dysrhythmias may interfere with timing the pump.

Minimally-invasive direct coronary artery bypass

*Copyright © Mometrix Media. You have been licensed one copy of this document for personal use only. Any other reproduction or redistribution is strictly prohibited. All rights reserved.*

Minimally-invasive direct coronary artery bypass (MIDCAB) applies a bypass graft on the beating heart through a 10-cm incision in the mid chest rather than midsternally, without using cardiopulmonary bypass. Because the incision must be over the bypass area, this procedure is suitable only for bypass of 1 or 2 coronary arteries. A small portion or rib is removed to allow access to the heart, and the internal mammary artery is used for grafting. Special instruments, such as a heart stabilizer, are used to limited movement of the heart during suturing. Surgery usually takes 2-3 hours and recovery time is decreased as patients have less pain. Because anastomosis is difficult on a beating heart, complications such as ischemia may occur during surgery so a cardiopulmonary bypass machine must be available. Early studies indicate that MIDCAB may provide longer-lasting relief than angioplasty for single vessel occlusion.

Port access coronary artery bypass graft

Port access coronary artery bypass graft is an alternative form of CABG that utilizes a number of small incisions (ports) along with cardiopulmonary bypass (CPB) and cardioplegia to do a video-assisted surgical repair. Usually, 3 or more incisions are required, with 1 in the femoral area to allow access to the femoral artery for a multipurpose catheter that is threaded through to the ascending aorta to return blood from the CPB, block the aorta with a balloon, provide cardioplegic solution, and vent air. Another catheter is threaded through the femoral vein to the right atrium to carry blood to the CPB. An incision is also needed for access to the jugular vein for catheters to the pulmonary artery and the coronary sinus. One to 3 thoracotomy incisions are made for insertion of video imaging equipment and instruments. While the midsternal incision is avoided, multiple incisions do pose the potential for possible morbidity.

Percutaneous transluminal coronary angioplasty

Percutaneous transluminal coronary angioplasty (PTCA) is an option for poor surgical candidates who have an acute MI or uncontrolled chest pain. This procedure is usually only done to increase circulation to the myocardium by breaking through an atheroma if there is collateral circulation. The patient receives IV sedation and local anesthesia. A hollow catheter (sheath) is inserted, usually from the femoral vein or artery, and fed through the vessels to the coronary arteries. When the atheroma is verified by fluoroscopy, a balloon-tipped catheter is fed over the sheath, and the balloon is inflated with a contrast agent to a specified pressure to compress the atheroma. The balloon may be inflated a number of times to ensure that residual stenosis is <20%. Laser angioplasty using the excimer laser is also used to vaporize plaque. **Stents** may be inserted during the angioplasty to maintain patency. Stents may be made of flexible plastic or wire mesh; they are typically placed over the catheter, which is inflated to expand the stent against the arterial wall.

**Directional coronary atherectomy**

Directional coronary atherectomy (DCA) is removal of an atheroma from an occluded coronary artery. The patient receives IV sedation and local anesthesia. This procedure may be more effective than angioplasty because it shaves an atheroma away instead of compressing it. Sometimes angioplasty is the first step in DCA if the vessel is too narrow for the DCA catheter and the last step if the tissue needs smoothing. The DCA catheter is a large balloon catheter usually inserted over a sheath through the femoral artery. The catheter includes an open window on 1 side of the balloon with a rotational cutting piston that shaves the atheroma with the plaque residue pushed inside the device for removal. The procedure may require 4-20 cuts, depending upon the extent of the plaque.

Rotational atherectomy:
A similar procedure is rotational atherectomy (ROTA), which uses a catheter with a diamond-

Copyright © Mometrix Media. You have been licensed one copy of this document for personal use only. Any other reproduction or redistribution is strictly prohibited. All rights reserved.

chip drill at the tip, rotating at 130,000-180,000 rpm, pulverizing the atheroma into microparticles.

<u>Transluminal extraction:</u>
Transluminal extraction catheter uses a motorized cutting head with a suction device for residue.

## Transmyocardial laser revascularization

Transmyocardial laser revascularization is done percutaneously or through a midsternal or thoracotomy incision. The patient receives general anesthesia (or local anesthesia and sedation for percutaneous procedure), but CPB is not needed unless this procedure is combined with coronary bypass surgery:

- Percutaneously, a fiberoptic catheter is positioned inside the ventricle and against the ischemic area. Laser bursts are used to cut 20-40 channels into but not through the myocardium. The laser burns create channels and stimulate an inflammatory response, which causes new blood vessels to form (angiogenesis), improving circulation to the myocardium and reducing ischemia and pain.
- Surgically, the catheter tip is positioned on the outside of the left ventricle rather than the inside while the heart is beating without bypass.

These procedures do not affect mortality but do reduce symptoms and increase tolerance to activity, improving the quality of life. Postoperative care for the percutaneous procedure is similar to that for PTCA; care for the surgical procedure is similar to that of coronary artery bypass graft (CABG).

## Postoperative care for cardiac surgeries

The postoperative care of cardiac surgery patients requires careful medical management:

- Cardiovascular support to maintain adequate cardiac output may require adjustment in heart rate, preload, afterload, and contractibility.

- Regulation of temperature following hypothermia that was induced during surgery requires warming, but not above 37°C.
- Bleeding must be monitored carefully and autotransfusion devices may be used to replace red blood cells.
- Chest tubes must be monitored for patency. "Milking" may cause less tissue damage than "stripping."
- Cardiac tamponade may occur if blood accumulates about the heart, requiring surgical intervention.
- Respiratory care includes early extubation (usually within 4-8 hours). Supplemental oxygen as needed.
- Neurological monitoring for *postcardiotomy delirium* (disorientation progressing to agitation, hallucinations, and paranoia).
- Wound infections may occur, especially if there is persistent fever. Diabetics may need insulin infusions to maintain glucose levels between 80-110 mg/dl to lower risk of infection.
- Hemoglobinuria can result from hemolysis and damage kidney tubules. Urine flow may be increased with Lasix® if <20-30 ml/hr or bloody.

## Heart transplant

Heart transplantation requires cardiopulmonary bypass (CPB) during the procedure with similar anesthetic consideration to other open heart procedures. After sternotomy, the pericardial sac is opened to expose the heart. If the donor heart is larger than the recipient's, the left pericardium, sparing the phrenic nerve, may be removed. The *orthotopic* procedure is most common: The posterior portion of the left and right atrium (with caval and pulmonary vein openings) is left for attachment of the new heart. The donor heart may be trimmed and is sutured to fit the remnants of the old heart. Once the donor heart is sutured, CPB is discontinued, and the heart is stimulated to begin contractions. Methylprednisolone is administered prior to removing aortic cross-clamp. Isoproterenol is

*Copyright © Mometrix Media. You have been licensed one copy of this document for personal use only. Any other reproduction or redistribution is strictly prohibited. All rights reserved.*

usually given before CPB is discontinued. The pulmonary artery catheter may be floated into position again after CPB to aid in evaluation. If right ventricular failure occurs from pulmonary hypertension, treatment with hyperventilation, prostaglandin, and nitric oxide may be used as well as a right ventricular assist device (RVAD).

Post-operative management:
Postoperative management of heart transplant patients is similar to that of other cardiac surgeries. *Treatments* include

- **Mechanical ventilation** is used initially, but respiratory care with adequate ventilation must be monitored constantly, especially if the donor heart was larger than the native heart, resulting in compression of the lungs.
- **Intravenous fluids** and various medications, such as sedatives and vasodilators, will be administered.
- **Prostaglandin** is continued for 1-2 days if used preoperatively to preclude rebound pulmonary hypertension.
- **Immunosuppression** therapy: anti-thymocyte globulin, azathioprine, cyclosporine or tacrolimus (Prograf®) may be used for immunosuppression as may corticosteroids (methylprednisolone). IV immunosuppressive drugs are given after surgery, but these are switched to oral medications when possible. Protocols are established at each institution and may vary. Medication doses are age-dependent.

The risk for rejection is the greatest in the first few months, and close follow up with regular, routine laboratory tests, including echocardiograms, chest x-rays, and blood tests, is necessary.

## Pulse oximetry

Pulse oximetry, continuous or intermittent, utilizes an external oximeter that attaches to the patient's finger or earlobe to measure arterial oxygen saturation ($SPO_2$), the percentage of hemoglobin that is saturated with oxygen. The oximeter also usually attaches to a machine that emits a beep with each heartbeat and indicates the current heart rate. Blood pressure (BP) monitoring is also done. The oximeter uses light waves to determine oxygen saturation ($SPO_2$). Oxygen saturation should be maintained >95%, although some patients with chronic respiratory disorders, such as chronic obstructive pulmonary disease (COPD) may have lower $SPO_2$. Results may be compromised by impaired circulation, excessive light, poor positioning, and nail polish. If $SPO_2$ falls, the oximeter should be repositioned, as incorrect position is a common cause of inaccurate readings. Oximetry is often used postsurgically and when patients are on mechanical ventilation. Oximeters do not provide information about carbon dioxide levels, so they cannot monitor carbon dioxide retention. Oximeters cannot differentiate between different forms of hemoglobin, so if hemoglobin has picked up carbon monoxide, the oximeter will not recognize that.

## Basic cardiac hemodynamics

Hemodynamics is based on the principle that fluid flows from areas of higher pressure to areas of lower pressure:

- **Systole:** Pressure rises in the ventricles, closing tricuspid and mitral (atrioventricular) valves, stopping flow from the atria and preventing backflow (regurgitation). Pressure forces the pulmonic and aortic valves (semilunar valves) open, sending blood into both the aorta and pulmonary artery. Early ventricular systolic pressure is high and then falls near the end of systole as the ventricles empty, lowering the pressure in the aorta and pulmonary artery, causing atrioventricular valves to close.
- **Diastole**: Ventricles are relaxed and atrioventricular valves open. Pressure in the atria is lower than in the venae cavas or pulmonary veins, pulling blood into the atria with some into the ventricles. An electrical impulse is generated in the Sino-atrial node (SA node), forcing the atria to contract, increasing the pressure and forcing more blood through the valves and into the

*Copyright © Mometrix Media. You have been licensed one copy of this document for personal use only. Any other reproduction or redistribution is strictly prohibited. All rights reserved.*

ventricles. This period is atrial systole and occurs near the end of ventricular diastole.

Cardiac output:
Cardiac output (CO) is the amount of blood pumped through the ventricles during a specified period. Normal cardiac output is about 5 liters per minute at rest for an adult. Under exercise or stress, this volume may multiply 3 or 4 times, with concomitant changes in the heart rate (HR) and stroke volume (SV). The basic formulation for calculating cardiac output is the heart rate (HR) per minute multiplied by the stroke volume (SV), which is the amount of blood pumped through the ventricles with each contraction. The stroke volume is controlled by preload, afterload, and contractibility.

$$CO = HR \times SV$$

The heart rate is controlled by the autonomic nervous system. Normally, if the heart rate decreases, stroke rate increases to compensate, but with cardiomyopathies, this may not occur, so bradycardia results in a sharp decline in cardiac output.

Preload and afterload:
Preload refers to the amount of elasticity in the myocardium at the end of diastole when the ventricles are filled to their maximum volume, and the stretch on the muscle fibers is the greatest. The preload value is based on the volume in the ventricles. The amount of preload (stretch) affects stroke volume because as stretch increases, the resultant contraction also increases (Frank-Starling Law). Preload may decrease because of dehydration, diuresis, or vasodilation. Preload may increase because of increased venous return, controlled fluid loss, transfusion, or intravenous fluids.
Afterload refers to the amount of systemic vascular resistance to left ventricular ejection of blood and pulmonary vascular resistance to right ventricular ejection of blood. Determinants of afterload include the size and elasticity of the great vessels and the functioning of the pulmonic and aortic valves. Afterload increases with hypertension, stenotic valves, and vasoconstriction.

Contractibility:
Contractibility is the amount of force exerted by the myocardium during contraction. It is directly related to both preload (elasticity) and afterload (systemic resistance). Many things affect contractibility:

- *Increased contractibility* may be due to changes in body chemistry or the sympathetic nervous system. Some drugs, such as digoxin and dopamine, also increase contractibility. This increase in contractibility results in increased stroke volume and cardiac output.
- *Decreased contractibility* may be due to hypoxemia and acidosis. Some drugs, such as beta-adrenergic blocking agents (atenolol), also decrease contractibility.

The heart can respond to the need for increased stroke volume (such as during exercise or periods of stress) by increasing preload through increasing venous return, increasing contractibility through stimulation of the sympathetic nervous system, and decreasing afterload with vasodilation. The *ejection fraction*, the percentage of end-diastolic blood ejected with each stroke (42% right ventricle, 50% left ventricle), can be used to determine contractibility because the ejection percentage decreases as contractibility decreases.

Perfusion and pulse pressure:
The perfusion pressure (measured by the mean arterial pressure – MAP) that is necessary may vary with different conditions and circumstances. The pulse pressure is the difference between systolic and diastolic pressures, and this can be an important indicator. For example, with a decrease in cardiac output, vasoconstriction takes place in the body's attempt to maintain the blood pressure. In this case, the MAP may remain unchanged, but the pulse pressure narrows. Necessary values for MAP include:
- >60 mm Hg to perfuse coronary arteries.
- 70-90 mm Hg to perfuse the brain and other organs, such as the kidneys, and to maintain cardiac patients and decrease the workload of the left ventricle.

*Copyright © Mometrix Media. You have been licensed one copy of this document for personal use only. Any other reproduction or redistribution is strictly prohibited. All rights reserved.*

- 90-110 to increase cerebral perfusion after neurosurgical procedures, such as carotid endarterectomy.

Patients should be assessed for changes in pulse pressure that may be precipitated by medications, such as diuretics that alter fluid volume.

Hemodynamic terms:
Cardiac output (CO) is the amount of blood pumped through the ventricles, usually calculated in liters per minute. Normal value at rest: 4-6 L/min.

Cardiac index (CI) is the cardiac output (CO) divided by the body surface area (BSA). This is essentially a measure of cardiac output tailored to the individual, based on height and weight, measured in liters/min per square meter of BSA. Normal value: 2.2-4.0 L/min/m$^2$.

Stroke volume (SV) is the amount of blood pumped through the left ventricle with each contraction, minus any blood remaining inside the ventricle at the end of systole. Normal values 60-70 ml. Formula:
- (CO in L/min) x (heart rate per minute) x (1000) = SV in ml.

Pulmonary vascular resistance (PVR) is the resistance in the pulmonary arteries and arterioles against which the right ventricle has to pump during contraction. It is the mean pressure in the pulmonary vascular bed divided by blood flow. If PVR increases, SV decreases. Normal value: 1.2-3.0 units or 100-250 dynes/sec/cm$^5$.

**Thoracic electrical bioimpedance monitoring**

Thoracic electrical bioimpedance monitoring is a non-invasive method of monitoring hemodynamics (CO, blood flow, contractility, preload and afterload, pulmonary artery pressure). Electrodes placed on the thorax measure changes in electrical output associated with the volume of blood through the aorta and its velocity. The monitor to which the electrodes are attached converts the signals to waveforms.

The heart rate is shown on an ECG monitor. The equipment calculates the cardiac output based on the heart rate and fluid volume. A typical bioimpedance monitor has 4 sets of bioimpedance electrodes and 3 ECG electrodes. Values for height, weight, and length of thorax are entered into the machine. Two (2) sets of bioimpedance electrodes are placed at the base of the neck bilaterally, and then 2 sets are placed on each side of the chest. The values for the distance between the neck electrodes and the chest electrodes (on the same side) must be measured and entered into the machine. ECG leads are placed where they consistently monitor the QRS signal (they may need to be moved to achieve this).

**Cardiac tamponade**

Cardiac tamponade occurs with pericardial effusion in which fluid accumulates in the pericardial sac, causing pressure against the heart. It may be a complication of trauma, pericarditis, cardiac surgery, or heart failure. About 50 ml of fluid normally circulates in the pericardial area to reduce friction, and a sudden increase in this volume can compress the heart causing a number of cardiac responses:
- Increased end-diastolic pressure in both ventricles.
- Decrease in venous return.
- Decrease in ventricular filling.

*Symptoms* may include a feeling of pressure or pain in the chest as well as dyspnea and pulsus paradoxus >10 mm Hg (systolic blood pressure heard during exhalation but not during inhalation). Beck's triad ($\uparrow$ central venous pressure with distended neck veins, muffled heart sounds, and hypotension) is commonly found. *Treatment* includes pericardiocentesis with large bore needle or surgical repair to control bleeding and relieve cardiac compression.

**Cardiogenic shock**

Cardiogenic shock in adults most often is secondary to myocardial infarction damage that

*Copyright © Mometrix Media. You have been licensed one copy of this document for personal use only. Any other reproduction or redistribution is strictly prohibited. All rights reserved.*

reduces the contractibility of the ventricles, interfering with the pumping mechanism of the heart, decreasing oxygen perfusion. Cardiogenic shock has 3 characteristics:

- Increased preload.
- Increased afterload.
- Decreased contractibility.

Together, these result in a decreased cardiac output and an increase in systemic vascular resistance (SVR) to compensate and protect vital organs. This results in an increase of afterload in the left ventricle with increased need for oxygen. As the cardiac output continues to decrease, tissue perfusion decreases, coronary artery perfusion decreases, fluid backs up, and the left ventricle fails to adequately pump the blood, resulting in pulmonary edema and right ventricular failure. *Symptoms* include:

- Hypotension with systolic BP <90 mm Hg.
- Tachycardia >100 beats/min with weak thready pulse and dysrhythmias.
- Decreased heart sounds.
- Chest pain.
- Tachypnea and basilar rales.
- Pallor.
- Cool, moist skin.

## Cardiomyopathy

Hypertrophic cardiomyopathy:
Hypertrophic cardiomyopathy (also known as asymmetric septal hypertrophy) is a rare genetic and occasionally idiopathic disorder that is often undetected until adolescence when the increasing symptoms become noticeable. With hypertrophic cardiomyopathy, the heart mass and size increase, especially with thickness along the septum, resulting in smaller ventricular capacity so that the ventricles fill less efficiently, and the atria have to work harder. This thickening may be asymmetrical. The disease may be nonobstructive or obstructive. The increased size of the septum may pull structures, such as the mitral valve, out of alignment, causing

some obstruction of the flow of blood through the valve to the aorta (idiopathic hypertrophic subaortic stenosis). The changes in the ventricles may result in increasing diastolic abnormalities, although systolic function is usually normal or high. When diagnosed in young people, the disease is often more severe than when it is diagnosed later in life.

Dilated cardiomyopathy:
Dilated cardiomyopathy, the most frequently occurring type of cardiomyopathy, occurs with an increase in the size of the ventricles (without a concomitant increase in hypertrophy of the ventricular muscle) as well as systolic dysfunction. The tissue loses elasticity, and areas of myocardial cells become necrotic. This loss in elasticity results in less blood being ejected during ventricular systole, so that during diastole, less blood is able to enter the partially-filled ventricles. This results in both an increase in pressure at the end of diastole and an increase in pulmonary pressure. As the ventricles stretch, the valves may be displaced, causing regurgitation. The poor blood flow can also cause thrombus formation and emboli. Many different conditions can cause dilated cardiomyopathy, including pregnancy, alcoholism, toxic compounds, autoimmune disease, and viral infections. Progress of the disease is often very slow, so diagnosis may be delayed until the disease is advanced and the patient suffers symptoms that require medical attention.

Restrictive cardiomyopathy:
Restrictive cardiomyopathy is the least common type of cardiomyopathy, but it is a common complication of heart transplants although, ironically, 1 of the treatments for the disorder is heart transplantation. The condition may be idiopathic or secondary. The disease is often related to amyloidosis, a condition in which the protein amyloid is deposited in the cells, but many times the cause of restrictive cardiomyopathy is unknown. While the heart

*Copyright © Mometrix Media. You have been licensed one copy of this document for personal use only. Any other reproduction or redistribution is strictly prohibited. All rights reserved.*

may be almost normal in size, the ventricular walls become increasingly fibrotic and rigid, so the ventricles cannot relax and fill adequately during diastole. As the disease progresses, the ventricles also are unable to contract effectively, reducing blood flow and increasing pulmonary and peripheral and systemic edema. Because there is no cure, early diagnosis and management of symptoms is important. The condition most commonly occurs in children but can affect young adults. Medical treatment includes the use of β-blockers to allow the ventricles to fill more effectively.

Arrhythmogenic right ventricular cardiomyopathy:
Arrhythmogenic right ventricular cardiomyopathy is an inherited (autosomal dominant and sometimes autosomal recessive) disease in which the myocardium of the right ventricle is slowly replaced with fibrotic and adipose tissue. While the condition begins in localized areas of the right ventricular muscle, eventually it can affect the left ventricular muscle as well. As the disease progresses, the right ventricle dilates and develops abnormalities of the ventricular walls, losing the ability to contract effectively. Dysrhythmias, such as right ventricular tachycardia develop. While many people can live with the disease with no or few symptoms, the disease may cause severe symptoms in others and may be the cause of sudden death in young athletes. It is reported more frequently in athletes than in other groups although a causative relationship is not believed. This diagnosis is usually made during the teens or early 20s when symptoms limit a young person's activities.

**Atrioventricular block**

First degree:
First degree atrioventricular (AV) block occurs when the atrial impulses are conducted through the AV node to the ventricles at a rate that is slower than normal. While the P and QRS are usually normal, the PR interval is >0.20 seconds, and the P:QRS ratio is 1:1. A narrow QRS complex indicates a conduction abnormality only in the AV node, but a widened QRS indicates associated damage to the bundle branches as well. *Chronic* first-degree block may be caused by fibrosis/sclerosis of the conduction system related to coronary artery disease, valvular disease, and cardiac myopathies but carries little morbidity. *Acute* first degree block, on the other hand, is of much more concern and may be related to digoxin toxicity, β-blockers, amiodarone, myocardial infarction, hyperkalemia, or edema related to valvular surgery. Incidence correlates with increasing age, and first-degree block is rare in young adults, although athletes have a higher rate (8.7%) than the elderly (5%).

Second degree:
Second degree AV block occurs when some of the atrial beats are blocked. Second degree AV block is further subdivided according to the patterns of block:
***Mobitz type I block (Wenckebach):*** Each atrial impulse in a group of beats is conducted at a lengthened interval until 1 fails to conduct (the PR interval progressively increases), so there are more P waves than QRS, but the shape and duration of the QRS complex is usually normal. The sinus node functions at a regular rate, so the P-P interval is regular, but the R-R interval usually shortens with each impulse. The P:QRS ratio varies, such as 3:2, 4:3, or 5:4. This type of block by itself usually does not cause significant morbidity unless associated with inferior wall myocardial infarction, during which a temporary pacemaker may be utilized.

***Mobitz type II block:*** Only some of the atrial impulses are conducted unpredictably through the AV node to the ventricles, and the block always occurs below the AV node in the bundle of His, the bundle branches, or the Purkinje fibers. The PR intervals are the same if impulses are conducted, but the QRS complex is usually widened. The P:QRS ratio varies 2:1, 3:1, and 4:1. Type II block is more dangerous than Type I

*Copyright © Mometrix Media. You have been licensed one copy of this document for personal use only. Any other reproduction or redistribution is strictly prohibited. All rights reserved.*

because it may progress to complete AV block and may produce Stokes-Adams syncope. Additionally, if the block is at the Purkinje fibers, there is no escape impulse. Usually a transcutaneous cardiac pacemaker and defibrillator should be at bedside. Symptoms may include chest pain if the heart block is precipitated by myocarditis or myocardial ischemia.

***2:1 block:*** Every other atrial impulse (P:QRS ratio of 2.1) is conducted through the AV node, and a surface ECG cannot differentiate between Type I and Type II.

Third degree:

With third degree AV block, there are more P waves than QRS with no clear relationship between them and an atrial rate that is 2-3 times the pulse rate, so the PR interval is irregular. If the SA node malfunctions, the AV node fires at a lower rate, and if the AV node malfunctions, the pacemaker site in the ventricles takes over at a bradycardic rate; thus, with complete AV block, the heart still contracts, but often ineffectually. With this type of block, the atrial P (sinus rhythm or atrial fibrillation) and the ventricular QRS (ventricular escape rhythm) are stimulated by different impulses, so there is AV dissociation. The heart may compensate at rest but can't keep pace with exertion. The resultant bradycardia may cause congestive heart failure, fainting, or even sudden death; usually conduction abnormalities slowly worsen. Symptoms include dyspnea, chest pain, and hypotension, which are treated with IV atropine. Transcutaneous pacing may be needed. Complete persistent AV block normally requires implanted pacemakers, usually dual chamber.

## Pacemakers

Pacemakers are used to stimulate the heart when the normal conduction system of the heart is defective. Pacemakers may be used temporarily or permanently implanted. While permanent pacemakers are commonly used to control chronic heart block, temporary pacemakers are more commonly found in the critical care setting. Temporary pacemakers may be used prophylactically or therapeutically to treat a cardiac abnormality. Clinical uses include

- To treat persistent dysrhythmias not responsive to medications.
- To increase cardiac output with bradydysrhythmia by increasing rate.
- To decrease ventricular or supraventricular tachycardia by "overdrive" stimulation of contractions.
- To treat secondary heart block caused by myocardial infarction, ischemia, and drug toxicity.
- To improve cardiac output after cardiac surgery.
- To provide diagnostic information through electrophysiology studies, which induce dysrhythmias for purposes of evaluation.
- To provide pacing when a permanent pacemaker malfunctions.

Types of pacemakers:

Pacemakers are used primarily for 3° atrioventricular block, sinus bradycardia, and atrioventricular block that occur after surgery. The parts of the pacemaker include 1 (unipolar) or 2 (bipolar) pacing leads that attach to the atrial or ventricular myocardium, or to the epicardium in some cases, to sense electrical impulses, leading to an implantable pulse generator (IPG) that contains a lithium battery and microprocessors for permanent pacemakers; temporary pacemakers are usually powered by 9-volt batteries in an external generator. The choice of single or double lead pacemakers depends upon the condition of the heart and whether the arrhythmias are atrial, ventricular, or both. There are different settings for pacemakers:

- ***Asynchronous*** is fixed-rate pacing.
- ***Synchronous*** is on-demand pacing that delivers an impulse if the pulse falls below a preset level.
- ***Dual chamber*** is AV sequential and delivers an impulse to the atrium and ventricle in sequence, allowing time for the ventricles to fill properly.

*Copyright © Mometrix Media. You have been licensed one copy of this document for personal use only. Any other reproduction or redistribution is strictly prohibited. All rights reserved.*

Complications:

Pacemakers are invasive foreign bodies and as such can cause a number of different complications:

- Infection, bleeding, or hematoma may occur at the entry site of leads for temporary pacemakers or at the subcutaneous area of implantation for permanent generators.
- Puncture of the subclavian vein or internal mammary artery may cause a hemothorax.
- The endocardial electrode may irritate the ventricular wall, causing ectopic beats or tachycardia.
- Dislodgement of transvenous lead may result in malfunction or perforation of the myocardium. This is 1 of the most common early complications.
- Dislocation of leads may result in phrenic nerve or muscle stimulation (which may be evidenced by hiccupping).
- Cardiac tamponade may result when epicardial wires of temporary pacing are removed.
- General malfunctioning of pacemaker may indicate dislodgement, dislocation, interference caused by electromagnetic fields, and the need for new batteries or generator.

## Cardiac dysrhythmias

Cardiac dysrhythmias, abnormal heart beats, in adults are frequently the result of damage to the conduction system during major cardiac surgery or as the result of a myocardial infarction.

Bradydysrhythmia are pulse rates that are abnormally slow:

- *Complete atrioventricular block (A-V block)* may be congenital or a response to surgical trauma.
- *Sinus bradycardia* may be caused by the autonomic nervous system or a response to hypotension and decrease in oxygenation.
- *Junctional/nodal rhythms* often occur in post-surgical patients when the absence of P wave is noted but heart rate and output usually

remain stable. Unless there is compromise, usually no treatment is necessary.

Tachydysrhythmia are pulse rates that are abnormally fast:

- *Sinus tachycardia* is often caused by illness, such as fever or infection.
- *Supraventricular tachycardia* (200-300 beats per minute [bpm]) may have a sudden onset and result in congestive heart failure.

Conduction irregularities are irregular pulses that often occur post-operatively and are usually not significant:

*Premature contractions* may arise from the atria or ventricles.

## Sinus bradycardia

There are 3 primary types of sinus node dysrhythmias: sinus bradycardia, sinus tachycardia, and sinus arrhythmia. Sinus bradycardia (SB) is caused by a decreased rate of impulse from the sinus node. The pulse and ECG usually appear normal except for a slower rate. SB is characterized by a regular pulse (<60 bpm) with P waves in front of QRS, which are usually normal in shape and duration. The PR interval is 0.12-0.20 seconds and the P:QRS ratio is 1:1. SB may be caused by a number of factors:

- Conditions that lower the body's metabolic needs, such as hypothermia or sleep.
- Medications such as calcium channel blockers and β-blockers.
- Vagal stimulation that may result from vomiting, suctioning, or defecating.
- ↑ Intracranial pressure.
- Myocardial infarction.

*Treatment* involves eliminating the cause if possible, such as changing medications. An atropine dose of 0.5-1.0 mg may be given IV to block vagal stimulation.

## Sinus tachycardia

Sinus tachycardia (ST) occurs when the sinus node impulse increases in frequency. ST is characterized by a regular pulse that is >100

*Copyright © Mometrix Media. You have been licensed one copy of this document for personal use only. Any other reproduction or redistribution is strictly prohibited. All rights reserved.*

bpm with P waves before QRS but sometimes part of the preceding T wave. QRS is usually of normal shape and duration but there may be consistent irregularity. The PR interval is 0.12-0.20 seconds and P:QRS ratio is 1:1. The rapid pulse decreases diastolic filling time and causes reduced cardiac output with resultant hypotension. Acute pulmonary edema may result from the decreased ventricular filling if untreated. ST may be caused by a number of factors:

- Acute blood loss.
- Shock.
- Anemia.
- Hypovolemia.
- Sinus arrhythmia.
- Heart failure (hypovolemic).
- Hypermetabolic conditions.
- Fever.
- Anxiety.
- Exertion/exercise.
- Medications, such as sympathomimetic drugs.

*Treatment* includes eliminating precipitating factors and prescribing calcium channel blockers and β-blockers to reduce heart rate.

## Sinus arrhythmia

Sinus arrhythmia (SA) results from irregular impulses from the sinus node, often paradoxical (increasing with inspiration and decreasing with expiration) because of stimulation of the vagal nerve during inspiration, although rarely causing a negative hemodynamic effect. These cyclic changes in the pulse during respiration are quite common in both children and young adults and often lessen with age, although SA may persist in some adults. Sinus arrhythmia can, in some cases, relate to heart or valvular disease and may be increased with vagal stimulation for suctioning, vomiting, or defecating. Characteristics of SA include a regular pulse of 50-100 bpm, P waves in front of QRS with duration and shape of QRS usually normal, PR interval of 0.12-0.20 seconds and P:QRS ratio of

1:1. Treatment is usually not necessary unless it is associated with bradycardia.

## Premature atrial contractions

There are 3 primary types of atrial dysrhythmias, including premature atrial contractions, atrial flutter, and atrial fibrillation. Premature atrial contractions (PAC) are essentially an extra beat precipitated by an electrical impulse to the atrium before the sinus node impulse. The extra beat may be caused by alcohol, caffeine, nicotine, hypervolemia, hypokalemia, hypermetabolic conditions, atrial ischemia or infarction. Characteristics include an irregular pulse because of extra P waves, shape and duration of QRS is usually normal but may be abnormal, PR interval remains between 0.12-0.20 seconds and P:QRS ratio is 1:1. PACs can occur in an essentially healthy heart and are not usually cause for concern unless they are frequent (>6/hr) and cause severe palpitations. In that case, atrial fibrillation should be suspected and may require antiarrhythmic drugs. In most cases, eliminating the cause (such as caffeine) helps to control the PACs.

## Atrial flutter

Atrial flutter (AF) occurs when the atrial rate is faster, usually 250-400 bpm, than the AV node conduction rate so that not all of the beats are conducted into the ventricles but are effectively blocked at the AV node. This prevents ventricular fibrillation, although some extra ventricular impulses may go through. AF is caused by the same conditions that cause atrial fibrillation: coronary artery disease, valvular disease, pulmonary disease, heavy alcohol ingestion, and cardiac surgery. AF is characterized by atrial rates of 250-400 bpm with ventricular rates of 75-150 bpm that are usually regular. P waves are saw-toothed (referred to as F waves), QRS shape and duration are usually normal, PR interval may be hard to calculate because of F waves, and the P:QRS ratio is 2-4:1. Symptoms include chest pain, dyspnea, and hypotension. Treatment includes:

- Cardioversion if condition is unstable.

*Copyright © Mometrix Media. You have been licensed one copy of this document for personal use only. Any other reproduction or redistribution is strictly prohibited. All rights reserved.*

- Medications to slow ventricular rate and conduction through AV node, e.g., Cardizem®, Calan®.
- Medications to convert to sinus rhythm, e.g., Corvert®, Cardioquin®, Norpace®, Cordarone®.

## Atrial fibrillation

Atrial fibrillation (Afib) is rapid, disorganized atrial beats that are ineffective in emptying the atria so that blood pools and can lead to thrombus formation and emboli. The ventricular rate increases with a decreased stroke volume, and cardiac output decreases with increased myocardial ischemia, resulting in palpitations and fatigue. Afib is caused by coronary artery disease, valvular disease, pulmonary disease, heavy alcohol ingestion, and cardiac surgery. Afib in characterized by very irregular pulse with atrial rate of 300-600 bpm and ventricular rate of 120-200 bpm, shape and duration of QRS is usually normal. Fibrillatory (F) waves are seen instead of P waves. The PR interval cannot be measured, and the P:QRS ratio is highly variable. Afib often converts to normal sinus rhythm within 24 hours, but cardioversion may be needed if Afib persists for >48 hours. Medications may include:
- For acute, Ibutilide:  procainamide, digoxin.
- To maintain rhythm:  quinidine, amiodarone.
- To control ventricular rate: β-blockers, calcium channel blockers, and verapamil.
- Anticoagulant therapy.

## Premature junctional contractions

The area around the AV node is the junction, and dysrhythmias that arise from that area are called junctional dysrhythmias. There are 3 main types: premature junctional contraction, junctional escape rhythm, and AV nodal reentry tachycardia. Ectopic beats spread an impulse in 2 directions:  a retrograde (backward) conduction to the atria (causing an inverted P wave) and an antegrade (forward) conduction to the ventricles (causing a normal QRS). The P wave may precede, be part of, or follow the QRS. Premature junctional contractions are similar to premature atrial contractions and generally require no treatment, although they may be an indication of digoxin toxicity. The ECG may appear basically normal with an early QRS complex that is normal in shape and duration. The P wave may precede, be part of, or follow the QRS. Significant symptoms related to premature junctional contractions are rare.

## Junctional escape rhythm

Junctional escape rhythm occurs when the AV node takes over as the pacemaker of the heart because the sinus node is depressed. This is caused by increased vagal tone or a block at the AV node that prevents sinus node impulses from being transmitted. While the sinus node normally sends impulses of 60-100 bpm, the AV node junction sends impulses of 40-60 bpm. Thus, junctional escape rhythm is characterized by a regular atrial/ventricular rate of 40-60 bpm and, a QRS complex of usual shape and duration. The P wave may be inverted or may be absent, hidden, or after the QRS. If the P wave precedes the QRS, the PR interval is <0.12 seconds. The P:QRS ratio is 1:1 or 0:1. The junctional escape rhythm is a protective mechanism preventing asystole with failure of the sinus node. While this rhythm is usually tolerated well, restoring a sinus rhythm is attempted by inserting a pacemaker in case AV failure occurs, leaving no backup system.

## AV nodal reentry tachycardia

AV nodal reentry tachycardia occurs when an impulse conducts to the area of the AV node, and the impulse is sent in a rapidly repeating cycle back to the same area and to the ventricles, resulting in a fast ventricular rate. The onset and cessation are usually rapid. AV nodal reentry tachycardia (also known as paroxysmal atrial tachycardia or supraventricular tachycardia if no P waves) is characterized by atrial rate of 150-250 bpm with ventricular rate of 75-250 bpm, P wave that is difficult to see or absent, QRS

*Copyright © Mometrix Media. You have been licensed one copy of this document for personal use only. Any other reproduction or redistribution is strictly prohibited. All rights reserved.*

complex that is usually normal, and a PR interval of <0.12 seconds if a P wave is present. The P:QRS ratio is 1-2:1. Precipitating factors include nicotine, caffeine, hypoxemia, and anxiety; also, underlying coronary artery disease and cardiomyopathy. Cardiac output may be decreased with a rapid heart rate, causing dyspnea, chest pain, and hypotension. Treatment may include:

- Vagal maneuvers (carotid sinus massage, gag reflex, holding breath.
- Medications (adenosine, verapamil, or diltiazem).
- Cardioversion if other methods are unsuccessful.

## Premature ventricular contractions

Premature ventricular contractions (PVCs) are those in which the impulse begins in the ventricles and conducts through them prior to the next sinus impulse. The ectopic QRS complexes may vary in shape, depending upon whether there is 1 (unifocal) or more (multifocal) sites stimulating the ectopic beats. PVCs usually cause no morbidity unless there is underlying cardiac disease or an acute MI. PVCs are characterized by an irregular heartbeat, QRS that is ≥0.12 seconds and oddly shaped, a P wave that may be absent or may precede or follow the QRS, a PR interval of <0.12 seconds if P wave is present, and P:QRS ratios of 0-1:1. Short-term therapy may include lidocaine, but PVCs are often not treated in otherwise healthy people. PVCs may be precipitated by caffeine, nicotine, or alcohol. Because PVCs may occur with any supraventricular dysrhythmia, the underlying rhythm (such as atrial fibrillation) must be noted as well as the PVCs.

## Ventricular tachycardia

Ventricular tachycardia (VT) is ≥3 PVCs in a row with a ventricular rate of 100-200 bpm. Ventricular tachycardia may be triggered by the same things as PVCs and is often related to underlying coronary artery disease, but the rapid rate of contractions make VT dangerous as the ineffective beats may render the person unconscious with no palpable pulse. A detectable rate is usually regular, and the QRS complex is ≥0.12 seconds and is usually abnormally shaped. The P wave may be undetectable, with an irregular PR interval if the P wave is present. The P:QRS ratio is often difficult to ascertain because of the absence of P waves. Treatment depends upon the degree of VT and the patient's tolerance and general condition. VT may convert spontaneously or may require cardioversion. Defibrillation is usually done as an emergency procedure if the patient is unconscious.

## Ventricular fibrillation

Ventricular fibrillation (VF) is a rapid, very irregular ventricular rate, such as >300 bpm, with no atrial activity observable on the ECG, caused by disorganized electrical activity in the ventricles. The QRS complex is not recognizable as the ECG shows irregular undulations. The causes are the same as the causes for ventricular tachycardia (VT), i.e., alcohol, caffeine, nicotine, underlying coronary disease, and VF may result if VT is not treated. It may also result from an electrical shock or congenital disorder, such as Brugada syndrome. VF is accompanied by lack of palpable pulse, audible pulse, and respirations and is immediately life threatening without defibrillation. After emergency defibrillation, the cause should be identified and limited. Antiarrhythmic medications, such as amiodarone, may be alternated with cardioversion in an attempt to convert the heart rhythm to normal. Mortality is high if VF occurs as part of a myocardial infarction.

## Ventricular escape rhythm

Ventricular escape rhythm (idioventricular) occurs when the Purkinje fibers below the AV node create an impulse. This may occur if the sinus node fails to fire, or if there is blockage at the AV node so that the impulse does not go through. Idioventricular rhythm is characterized by a regular ventricular rate of 20-40 bpm. Rates >40 are called accelerated idioventricular rhythm. The QRS complex has a very abnormal shape, and the duration is ≥0.12 seconds. The

*Copyright © Mometrix Media. You have been licensed one copy of this document for personal use only. Any other reproduction or redistribution is strictly prohibited. All rights reserved.*

low ventricular rate causes a decrease in cardiac output, often making the patient lose consciousness. In some cases, symptoms may be few, but bed rest is required to decrease cardiac workload. *Treatment* may include defibrillation, IV atropine, and vasopressors. Transcutaneous pacing may be required as an emergency intervention. The underlying cause of the idioventricular rhythm should be identified and treated to prevent recurrence.

### Ventricular asystole

Ventricular asystole is the absence of audible heartbeat, palpable pulse, and respirations, a condition often referred to as "flat lining" or "cardiac arrest." While the ECG may show some P waves initially, the QRS complex is absent although there may be an occasional QRS "escape beat." Cardiopulmonary resuscitation is required with intubation for ventilation and establishment of an intravenous line for fluids. Without immediate treatment, the patient will suffer from severe hypoxia and brain death within minutes. Identifying the cause is critical for the patient's survival and could include hypoxia, acidosis, electrolyte imbalance, hypothermia, or drug overdose. Even with immediate treatment, the prognosis is poor, and ventricular asystole is often a sign of impending death. Additional treatment may include transcutaneous pacing and IV epinephrine, repeated at intervals of 3-5 minutes, followed by atropine each time.

### Cardioversion

Cardioversion is a timed electrical stimulation to the heart to convert a tachydysrhythmia (such as atrial fibrillation) to a normal sinus rhythm. Usually, anticoagulation therapy is done for at least 3 weeks before elective cardioversion to reduce the risk of emboli, and digoxin is discontinued for at least 48 hours before cardioversion. During the procedure, the patient is usually sedated and/or anesthetized. Electrodes in the form of gel-covered paddles or pads are positioned in the left chest and left back (in front of and behind the heart) and connected by leads to a computerized ECG and a cardiac monitor/defibrillator. The defibrillator is synchronized with the ECG so that the electrical current is delivered during ventricular depolarization (QRS). The timing must be precise in order to prevent ventricular tachycardia or ventricular fibrillation. Sometimes, drug therapy is used in conjunction with cardioversion; for example, antiarrhythmics (Cardizem®, Cordarone®) may be given before the procedure to slow the heart rate.

### Emergency defibrillation

Emergency defibrillation is done to treat acute ventricular fibrillation or ventricular tachycardia when there is no audible or palpable pulse. A higher voltage is generally used for defibrillation than for cardioversion. This higher voltage causes depolarization of myocardial cells, which can then repolarize to regain a normal sinus rhythm. Defibrillation delivers an electrical discharge usually through paddles applied to both sides of the chest. Defibrillation may be repeated, usually up to 3 times, at increasing voltage, but if the heart has not regained a sinus rhythm by then, cardiopulmonary resuscitation and advanced life support is required. Medications, such as epinephrine or vasopressin, may be administered, and cardiopulmonary resuscitation continued for 1 minute, after which defibrillation is again attempted. Additional medications, such as Cordarone®, magnesium, or procainamide, may be necessary if there are persistent ventricular dysrhythmias. *Automated external defibrillators* (AEDs) are frequently used by first responders and emergency personnel to provide defibrillation.

### Automatic implantable cardioverter defibrillator

The automatic implantable cardioverter defibrillator (AICD) is similar to the pacemaker and is implanted in the same way with 1 or more leads to the ventricular myocardium or the epicardium, but it is used to control tachycardia and/or fibrillation. Severe tachycardia may be

*Copyright © Mometrix Media. You have been licensed one copy of this document for personal use only. Any other reproduction or redistribution is strictly prohibited. All rights reserved.*

related to electrical disturbances, cardiomyopathy, or postoperative response to repair of congenital disease. In some cases, it is not responsive to medications. When the pulse reaches a certain preset rate, the device automatically provides a small electrical impulse to the atrial or ventricular myocardium to slow the heart. If fibrillation occurs, a higher energy shock is delivered. It takes 5-15 seconds for the device to detect abnormalities in the pulse rate, and because more than 1 shock may be required, the patient may faint before the procedure becomes effective. Some devices can function as both a pacemaker and an ICD, which is especially important for those who have episodes of both bradycardia and tachycardia.

## Heart failure

Heart failure (HF) (formerly congestive heart failure) is a cardiac disease that includes disorders of contractions (systolic dysfunction) or filling (diastolic dysfunction) or both and may include pulmonary, peripheral, or systemic edema. The most common causes are coronary artery disease, systemic or pulmonary hypertension, cardiomyopathy, and valvular disorders. The incidence of chronic heart failure correlates with age. There are 2 main types of HF: systolic and diastolic. HF is classified according to *symptoms* and prognosis:

- *Class I:* The patient is essentially asymptomatic during normal activities with no pulmonary congestion or peripheral hypotension. There is no restriction on activities, and prognosis is good.
- *Class II:* Symptoms appear with physical exertion but are usually absent at rest, resulting in some limitations of activities of daily life (ADLs). Slight pulmonary edema may be evident by basilar rales. Prognosis is good.
- *Class III:* Obvious limitations of ADLs and discomfort on any exertion. Prognosis is fair.
- *Class IV:* Symptoms at rest. Prognosis is poor.

Chronic heart failure:
Chronic heart failure (HF) develops more slowly than acute HF with the myocardium damaged by lack of adequate oxygenation and nutrition so that the myocardial cells begin to die, creating areas of necrosis. These in turn, stimulate the production of fibroblasts that replace cells with deposits of collagen, creating a fibrotic resistant myocardium. Existing myocytes increase in size but lose strength. There is cardiac dilation and increasing vascular resistance (afterload).

Acute heart failure:
Acute heart failure can occur with sudden onset, with the body attempting to compensate for circulatory malfunction by protecting blood flow to vital organs. There is an increase in the contractibility of the myocardium but peripheral vasoconstriction. Fluid and sodium are retained to control hypotension. However, the increased contractibility and heart rate produce a need for oxygen beyond that available, leading to a physiologic response that results in tissue necrosis, cardiotoxicity, pulmonary edema, and organ failure:

- *Capillary hypertension* decreases oncotic pressure and results in vasodilation and increased loss of fluid from the plasma to the interstitial fluid, resulting in pulmonary edema.
- *Capillary hypotension* results in increased oncotic pressure and pulls fluid back into the plasma, a result of shock.

Management of acute heart failure:
Acute heart failure is characterized by impairment of gas exchange and decreased cardiac output because of changes in preload, contractibility, and heart rhythm. Patients may also suffer from anxiety, decreased activity tolerance, and disturbances in sleep patterns. Medical management is aimed at increasing cardiac function, providing support, and monitoring treatment.
*Treatment* may include:

- Careful monitoring of fluid balance and weight to determine changes in fluid retention.
- Low sodium diet.

*Copyright © Mometrix Media. You have been licensed one copy of this document for personal use only. Any other reproduction or redistribution is strictly prohibited. All rights reserved.*

- Restriction of activity.
- Medications may include diuretics, vasodilators, or angiotensin converting enzyme (ACE) inhibitors to decrease the heart's workload. Digoxin may be given to increase contractibility.
- Anticoagulant therapy if distended atria, enlarged ventricles, or atrial fibrillation are present, in order to decrease the danger of thromboembolia.

Patient education is an important component of heart failure management in order to prevent recurrence. The patient should be an active participant in planning care as the acute condition stabilizes.

Systolic heart failure:
Systolic heart failure is the typical "left-sided" failure and reduces the amount of blood ejected from the ventricles during contraction (↓ ejection fraction), stimulating the sympathetic nervous system to produce epinephrine and norepinephrine to support the myocardium. However, this eventually causes down regulation in which beta and adrenergic receptor sites are destroyed, causing further myocardial damage. Because of reduced perfusion, the kidneys produce renin, which promotes angiotensin I, which is converted into angiotensin II, a vasoconstrictor, by the blood vessels. This in turn stimulates production of aldosterone, causing sodium and fluid retention. The end result of these processes is an increase in preload and afterload, increasing the workload on the heart, especially the ventricles. The heart muscle begins to lose contractibility, and blood begins to pool in the ventricles, stretching the myocardium and enlarging the ventricles (ventricular remodeling). The heart compensates by thickening the muscle (hypertrophy) without an adequate increase in capillary blood supply because of the vasoconstriction of the coronary arteries, leading to ischemia.

Diastolic heart failure:
Diastolic heart failure may be difficult to differentiate from systolic heart failure based on clinical symptoms, which are similar. With diastolic heart failure, the myocardium is unable to sufficiently relax to facilitate filling of the ventricles. This may be the end result of systolic heart failure as myocardial hypertrophy stiffens the muscles, and the causes are similar. Diastolic heart failure is more common in females >75. Typically, intracardiac pressures at rest are within normal range but increase markedly on exertion. Because the relaxation of the heart is delayed, the ventricles do not expand enough for the fill-volume, and the heart cannot increase stroke volume during exercise, so *symptoms* (dyspnea, fatigue, pulmonary edema) are often pronounced on exertion. Ejection fractions are usually >40%-50% with increase in left ventricular end-diastolic pressure (LVEDP) and decrease in left ventricular end-diastolic volume (LVEDV).

**Hypertensive crises**

Hypertensive crises are marked elevations in blood pressure that can cause severe organ damage if left untreated. Hypertensive crises may be related to primary or secondary hypertension, which may result from kidney or endocrine disorders. Other diseases that may precipitate hypertensive crises include dissection of an aortic aneurysm, pulmonary edema, CNS disorders (subarachnoid hemorrhage, stroke), eclampsia, and failure to take medications properly. There are 2 classifications:
- ***Hypertensive emergency*** occurs when acute hypertension (1.5 x the 95th percentile), usually >120 mm Hg diastolic, must be treated immediately to lower blood pressure in order to prevent damage to vital organs, such as the heart, brain, or kidneys.
- ***Hypertensive urgency*** occurs when acute hypertension must be treated within a few hours, but the vital organs are not in immediate danger.
  Blood pressure is lowered more slowly to avoid hypotension, ischemia of vital organs, or failure of autoregulation.
  o   1/3 reduction in 6 hours.
  o   1/3 reduction in next 24 hours.

Copyright © Mometrix Media. You have been licensed one copy of this document for personal use only. Any other reproduction or redistribution is strictly prohibited. All rights reserved.

o   1/3 reduction over days 2-4.

Treatment options:

Hypertensive crisis may be managed by a variety of different medications, depending upon the cause and whether the hypertension is an emergency or urgency. In some cases, medications may be combined. Patients with hypertensive emergency receive IV medications and oxygen. Medications include:

- Initial: Sodium nitroprusside (Nipride®) for fast-acting vasodilation.
- Short acting β-blockers (labetalol, esmolol) for dissecting aortic aneurysm.
- ACE inhibitors (enalaprilat) for heart failure.
- Nitroglycerine for chest pain.
- Dopamine-receptor agonist (fenoldopam) for renal disease to increase circulation to kidneys.
- Hydralazine for eclampsia.
- Calcium channel blocker (nicardipine) CNS disorders.
- Enalaprilat and labetalol for CNS disorders.
- Alpha-blocker (phentolamine) for pheochromocytoma.
- Diuretics, such as Lasix® and bumetanide to reduce edema.

Continuous monitoring of BP must be done and patient observed for hypotension cause by treatment. If the patient had a stroke, thrombolytic therapy (t-PA), should not be given if the systolic BP is >185 mm Hg and/or the diastolic BP is >110 mm Hg.

## Peripheral vascular insufficiency

Peripheral vascular insufficiency includes both arterial and venous disease:

- **Peripheral arterial disease (PAD)** involves the aorta, its branches, arteries, and arterioles. Peripheral arterial disease includes occlusion of the arteries of the lower extremities from atherosclerosis, resulting in severe pain and ischemia. The arteries most often affected by PAD are the femoral, the popliteal, the distal aorta and the iliac arteries. PAD is characterized by intermittent claudication, tissue changes, and ulcerations.
- **Peripheral venous insufficiency** results from defective valves in the deep and/or superficial veins of the lower extremities. Valvular defects may be related to damage, thrombus formation, or congenital weakness, but the result is a reflux of blood backwards. If the superficial veins are involved, the deep veins are normal, but the superficial veins become dilated (varicose veins). If the deep veins are involved because of deep vein thrombosis, there is an increase in pressure in the extremity.

| Arterial vs. venous insufficiency | | |
|---|---|---|
| **Characteristic** | **Arterial** | **Venous** |
| **Type of pain** | Ranges from inter-mittent claudication to severe constant. | Aching and cramping. |
| **Pulses** | Weak or absent. | Present. |
| **Skin of extremity** | Rubor on dependency but pallor of foot on elevation. Skin pale, shiny, and cool with loss of hair on toes and foot. Nails thick and ridged. | Brownish discoloration (hemosiderin) around ankles and anterior tibial area. Lipodermatosclerosis, varicosities, and/or venous dermatitis evident. |
| **Ulcers** | Pain, deep, circular, often necrotic ulcers on toe tips, toe webs, heels, or other pressure areas. | Varying degrees of pain in superficial, irregular ulcers on medial or lateral malleolus and sometimes the anterior tibial area. |
| **Extremity edema** | Minimal. | Moderate to severe. |

## Venous thromboembolism

Venous thromboembolism (VTE) **is** a condition that includes both deep vein thrombosis (DVT) and pulmonary emboli (PE). VTE may be

*Copyright © Mometrix Media. You have been licensed one copy of this document for personal use only. Any other reproduction or redistribution is strictly prohibited. All rights reserved.*

precipitated by invasive procedures, lack of mobility, and inflammation, so it is a common complication in acute/critical care units. Virchow's triad comprises common risk factors: blood stasis, injury to endothelium, and hypercoagulability. Some patients may be initially asymptomatic, but *symptoms* may include:

- Aching or throbbing pain.
- Positive Homan's sign (pain in calf when foot is dorsiflexed).
- Erythema and edema.
- Dilation of vessels.
- Cyanosis.

*Diagnosis* may be made by ultrasound and/or D-dimer test, which test the serum for cross-linked fibrin derivatives. Computed tomography (CT) scan, pulmonary angiogram, and ventilation-perfusion lung scan may be used to diagnose pulmonary emboli. Prophylaxis is very important, but once diagnosed; *treatment* involves bed rest, elevation of affected limb, anticoagulation therapy, and analgesics. Elastic stockings should be worn when the patient begins ambulating.

## Transcutaneous oxygen pressure measurement

Transcutaneous oxygen pressure measurement (TCPO$_2$) is a non-invasive test that measures dermal oxygen, showing effectiveness of oxygen in the skin and tissues. Contact gel and electrodes are applied to the lower extremities to determine variations in oxygen tension. The electrodes are placed in special fixation rings attached to the skin to prevent environment air from affecting the readings, and then the skin is heated to increase blood flow. Two or 3 different sites should be tested to give a more accurate demonstration of oxygenation. This test is used for a number of purposes:

- Determining if there is enough oxygen transport for effective hyperbaric oxygen therapy treatments.
- Determining the degree of oxygenation and peripheral vascular disease.

- Establishing the degree of hypoxia in venous diseases.
- Identifying the optimum site for amputation of severely hypoxic limbs.

Test results:

- >40 mm Hg adequate oxygenation for healing.
- 20-40 mm Hg equivocal finding.
- <20 mm Hg marked ischemia, affecting healing.

## Maximizing perfusion

The primary focus of pharmacologic measures to maximize perfusion is to reduce the risk of thromboses:

- **Antiplatelet agents**, such as aspirin, Ticlid®, and Plavix®, interfere with the function of the plasma membrane, interfering with clotting. These agents are ineffective to treat clots but prevent clot formation.
- **Vasodilators** may divert blood from ischemic areas, but some may be indicated, such as Pietal®, which dilates arteries and decreases clotting and is used for control of intermittent claudication.
- **Antilipemic**, such as Zocor® and Questran®, slow progression of atherosclerosis.
- **Hemorheologics**, such as Trental®, reduce fibrinogen, reducing blood viscosity and rigidity of erythrocytes; however, clinical studies show limited benefit. It may be used for intermittent claudication.
- **Analgesics** may be necessary to improve quality of life. Opioids may be needed in some cases.
- **Thrombolytics** (streptokinase) may be injected into a blocked artery under angiography to dissolve clots.
- **Anticoagulants**, such as Coumadin® and Lovenox®, prevent blood clots from forming.

## Arterial insufficiency and ulcers

Surgical/vascular interventions:
The goals of managing arterial insufficiency and ulcers are to improve perfusion and save the

*Copyright © Mometrix Media. You have been licensed one copy of this document for personal use only. Any other reproduction or redistribution is strictly prohibited. All rights reserved.*

limb, but lifestyle changes and medications may be insufficient. There are a number of indications for surgical intervention:

- Poor healing prognosis includes those with ankle brachial index (ABI) <0.5 because their perfusion is severely compromised.
- Failure to respond to conservative treatment (medications and lifestyle changes) even with an ABI >0.5.
- Intolerable pain, such as with severe intermittent claudication, that is incapacitating and limits the patient's ability to work or carry out activities. Rest pain is an indication that medical treatment is insufficient.
- Limb-threatening condition, such as severe ischemia with increasing pain at rest, infection, and/or gangrene. Infection can cause a wound to deteriorate rapidly.

Surgical intervention is indicated only for those patients with patent distal vessels as demonstrated by radiologic imaging procedures.

## Peripheral vascular surgery

Surgical/vascular surgery for treatment of severe arterial insufficiency includes 3 different types of procedures:

- **Bypass graft** in which a section of the saphenous vein or an upper extremity vein is harvested to use to bypass damaged arteries and supply blood to distal vessels. Because veins have valves, they must be reversed or stripped of valves prior to attachment. Synthetic grafts are also sometimes used, but they have a much higher failure rate.
- **Angioplasty** can be used if disease is not extensive (>10 cm in length), but arteries must be large enough to accommodate the procedure safely. Initial results are good but long-term rates have been less positive although the use of anticoagulants improves success rates.
- **Amputation** is the procedure that treatment tries to avoid, but it is sometimes required if ischemia is irreversible or if there is severe necrosis and infection that is life threatening.

## Pulmonary edema

Pulmonary edema occurs when excess fluid enters the pulmonary interstitium and alveoli because of increased pulmonary capillary pressure combined with decrease in the oncotic pressure, mechanical or physiologic damage to the capillary-alveolar membrane, or obstruction of the lymphatic drainage system:

- Mitral stenosis reduces the flow of blood to the left ventricle. Pressure in the left atrium increases to overcome resistance, resulting in enlargement of the left atrium and increased pressure in the pulmonary veins and capillaries of the lung.
- Tachycardia and/or atrial fibrillation may reduce blood flow to the left ventricle, resulting in increased atrial and pulmonary pressure.
- Left ventricular dysfunction reduces cardiac output and fluid backs up into the lungs, increasing the capillary pressure.

The increased pressure results in increased capillary vasodilation and fluid flows into the interstitium. Initially, lymphatic drainage increases to compensate but becomes overwhelmed as fluid accumulates. When the interstitium becomes engorged, the fluid crosses the alveolar membranes, and the alveoli cannot function, resulting in decreased gas exchange and hypoxemia.

Cardiac-related pulmonary edema:
Acute cardiac-related pulmonary edema may result from MI, chronic HF, volume overload, ischemia, or mitral stenosis. *Symptoms* include severe dyspnea, cough with blood-tinged frothy sputum, cyanosis, and diaphoresis. Patients have obvious wheeze with rales and rhonchi present throughout lung fields. *Diagnosis* is by auscultation, chest x-ray, and echocardiogram. *Treatment* includes:

- Sitting position with oxygen by mask to achieve $PO_2$ >60%.
- Non-invasive pressure support ventilation or endotracheal intubation and mechanical ventilation, depending upon severity of condition.

- 28 -

*Copyright © Mometrix Media. You have been licensed one copy of this document for personal use only. Any other reproduction or redistribution is strictly prohibited. All rights reserved.*

- Morphine sulfate 2-8 mg (IV for severe cases), repeated every 2-4 hours as needed.
- IV diuretics (furosemide ≥40 mg or bumetanide ≥1 mg) to provide venous dilation and diuresis.
- Nitrates, such as sublingual (SL) nitroglycerine or isosorbide, topical nitroglycerine, or IV nitrates, or IV nesiritide as a bolus with an infusion.
- Inhaled β-adrenergic agonists or aminophylline for bronchospasm.

## Ruptured or dissecting aneurysm

An aortic aneurysm occurs when a weakness in the wall of the aorta causes a ballooning dilation of the wall of the aorta. There are a number of types:
- **False** is caused by a hematoma that may pulsate and erode the wall of the vessel.
- **True bulging** involves 1-3 layers of the vessel wall.
- **Fusiform** is a symmetric bulging about the entire circumference of the vessel.
- **Saccular** is a ballooning on 1 side of the vessel wall.
- **Dissecting** splits the layers of the wall, usually caused by an expanding hematoma.

Aneurysms may result from infections or other trauma although atherosclerosis is the most common cause for both thoracic and abdominal aortic aneurysms. About 1/3 of thoracic aneurysms (often dissecting) rupture, so surgical repair is indicated. Abdominal aneurysms may remain stable for years, so surgery may be delayed for those at risk until the aneurysm is 5 cm wide.

Classification:
A dissecting aortic aneurysm occurs when the wall of the aorta is torn and blood flows between the layers of the wall, dilating and weakening it until it risks rupture (a condition with 90% mortality). Aortic aneurysms are more than twice as common in men as women, but women have a higher mortality rate, possibly because they are often older. Different classification systems are used to describe the type and degree of dissection. Common classifications include:
*DeBakey classification* using anatomic location as the focal point:
- *Type I* begins in the ascending aorta but may spread to include the aortic arch and the descending aorta (60%). This is also considered a proximal lesion or Stanford type A.
- *Type II* is restricted to the ascending aorta (10%-15%). This is also considered a proximal lesion or Stanford type A.
- *Type III* is restricted to the descending aorta (25%-30%). This is considered a distal lesion or Stanford type B.

Types I and II are thoracic and type III is abdominal.

Management:
Once a dissecting aortic aneurysm (thoracic or abdominal) is identified and the type is determined, both medical management and surgical repair may be indicated:
- *Anti-hypertensives* to reduce systolic BP, such as β-blockers (esmolol) or alpha-β-blocker combinations (labetalol) to reduce the force of the blood as it leaves the ventricle to reduce pressure against aortic wall. IV vasodilators (sodium nitroprusside) may also be needed.
- *Intubation and ventilation* may be required if the patient is hemodynamically unstable.
- *Analgesia/sedation* to control anxiety and pain.
- *Diagnostic tests*, such as CT, magnetic resonance imaging (MRI), transthoracic echocardiogram, and transesophageal echocardiograms may be needed.

*Type I and II* aneurysms are usually repaired surgically because of the danger of *rupture and cardiac tamponade.*
*Type III (abdominal)* aneurysms are often followed medically and the surgery delayed until the aneurysm is >5 cm, at which time either abdominal surgical repair or endoluminal stent may be done.

*Copyright © Mometrix Media. You have been licensed one copy of this document for personal use only. Any other reproduction or redistribution is strictly prohibited. All rights reserved.*

## Abdominal aortic aneurysm

About 90% of abdominal aortic aneurysms occur below the renal arteries, but aneurysms are not usually palpable until they reach 5 cm/diameter, so they may be found incidentally. Patients may have had mild constant or intermittent pain, but the rupture results in severe abdominal pain, hypotension, and a palpable mass. About 50% of patients die with rupture. Elective repair is usually advised for aneurysms >5.5 cm or those that are rapidly expanding. Ultrasound and CT are used for diagnosis, with CT with contrast to show vasculature. There are 2 types of surgical repair:

- *Open:* An abdominal incision is made with dissection of damaged aorta and a graft is sutured in place. Aortic blood flow must be interrupted with CPB during this procedure.
- *Endovascular:* A stent graft is fed through the arteries to line the aorta and exclude the aneurysm.

Complications include myocardial infarction, renal injury, and GI hemorrhage, which may occur up to years after surgery. Endo-leaks can occur with a stent graft, increasing the risk of rupture.

## Thoracic aortic aneurysm

Thoracic aortic aneurysms are usually related to atherosclerosis but may also result from Marfan syndrome, Ehlers-Danlos disease, and connective tissue disorders. The aneurysms are often asymptomatic but may cause substernal pain, back pain, dyspnea, and/or stridor (from pressure on the trachea), cough, distention of neck veins, and edema of neck and arms. Rupture usually does not allow time for emergent repair, so identifying and correcting the condition before rupture is essential. Diagnosis is often made with x-ray or CT. Cardiac catheterization and echocardiogram may also be needed. Surgery is indicated for aneurysms ≥6 cm. Endovascular grafting is routinely done for aneurysms of the descending thoracic aorta. Open surgical repair is required for the ascending aorta or arch, but these surgeries are much more dangerous with higher rates of morbidity and mortality than for abdominal aorta repair. There is a 4% occurrence of paraplegia with thoracic aorta aneurysm repair and an increased risk of stroke.

## Mitral stenosis

Mitral stenosis is caused by an autoimmune response to rheumatic fever leading to vegetative growths on the mitral valve. It can also be caused by infective endocarditis or lupus erythematosus. Over time, the leaflets thicken and calcify, and the commissures (junctions) fuse, decreasing the size of the valve opening. Mitral stenosis reduces the flow of blood from the left atrium to the left ventricle. Pressure in the left atrium increases to overcome resistance, resulting in enlargement of the left atrium and increased pressure in the pulmonary veins and capillaries of the lung. *Symptoms* of exertional dyspnea usually occur when the valve is 50% occluded. There are 3 mechanisms by which mitral stenosis causes pulmonary hypertension:

- Increased left atrial pressure causing backward increase in pressure of pulmonary veins.
- Hypertrophy and pulmonary artery constriction resulting from reactive left atrial and pulmonary venous hypertension.
- Thrombotic/embolitic damage to pulmonary vasculature.

*Treatment* includes drugs to control arrhythmias and hypertension, balloon valvuloplasty, and mitral valve replacement.

## Mitral valve regurgitation

Mitral valve regurgitation may occur with mitral stenosis or independently. It can result from damage caused by rheumatic fever, myxomatous degeneration caused by a genetic defect in the valvular collagen, infective endocarditis, collagen vascular disease (Marfan's syndrome) or cardiomyopathy. Hypertrophy and dilation of the left ventricle may cause displacement of the leaflets and dilation of the valve. Regurgitation occurs when the mitral valve fails to close

*Copyright © Mometrix Media. You have been licensed one copy of this document for personal use only. Any other reproduction or redistribution is strictly prohibited. All rights reserved.*

completely so that there is backflow into the left atrium from the left ventricle during systole, decreasing cardiac output. There are 3 phases:

- **Acute** may occur with rupture of chordae tendineae or papillary muscle causing sudden left ventricular flooding and overload.
- **Chronic compensated** results in enlargement of the left atrium to decrease filling pressure and hypertrophy of the left ventricle to maintain stroke volume and cardiac output.
- **Chronic decompensated** occurs when the left ventricle fails to compensate for the volume overload so that stroke volume and cardiac output decrease.

## Aortic stenosis

Aortic stenosis is a stricture (narrowing) of the aortic valve that controls the flow of blood from the left ventricle, causing the left ventricular wall to thicken as it increases pressure to overcome the valvular resistance, increasing afterload, and increasing the need for blood supply from the coronary arteries. Aortic stenosis may result from a birth defect or childhood rheumatic fever, and it tends to worsen over the years as the heart grows. *Symptoms* include:

- Chest pain on exertion and intolerance of exercise.
- Heart murmur.
- Hypotension on exertion may be associated with sudden fainting.
- Sudden death can occur.
- Tachycardia with faint pulse.
- Poor appetite.
- Increased risk for bacterial endocarditis and coronary insufficiency.
- Increases in mitral regurgitation and secondary pulmonary hypertension.

*Treatment* includes:

- Balloon valvuloplasty to dilate valve non-surgically.
- Surgical repair of valve or replacement of valve, depending upon the extent of stricture.

## Pulmonic stenosis

Pulmonic stenosis is a stricture of the pulmonic valve that controls the flow of blood from the right ventricle to the lungs, resulting in right ventricular hypertrophy as the pressure increases in the right ventricle and decreased pulmonary blood flows. The condition may be asymptomatic or symptoms may not be evident until adulthood, depending upon the severity of the defect. Pulmonic stenosis may be associated with a number of other heart defects. *Symptoms* of pulmonic stenosis can include:

- Loud heart murmur.
- Congestive heart murmur.
- Mild cyanosis.
- Cardiomegaly.
- Angina.
- Dyspnea.
- Fainting.
- Increased risk of bacterial endocarditis.

*Treatment* includes:

- Balloon valvuloplasty to separate the cusps of the valve for children.
- Surgical repair includes the cardiopulmonary bypass pulmonary valvotomy for older children and adults.

## Electrocardiogram

The electrocardiogram (ECG) provides a graphic representation of the electrical activity of the heart. It is indicated for chest pain, dyspnea, syncope, acute coronary syndrome, pulmonary embolism, and possible MI. The standard 12-lead ECG gives a picture of electrical activity from 12 perspectives through the placement of 10 body leads:

- 4 limb leads are placed distally on the wrists and ankles (but may be placed more proximally, if necessary).
- Precordial leads:
  - V1: right sternal border at 4th intercostal space.
  - V2: left sternal border at 4th intercostal space.
  - V3: Midway between V2 and V4.

*Copyright © Mometrix Media. You have been licensed one copy of this document for personal use only. Any other reproduction or redistribution is strictly prohibited. All rights reserved.*

- o V4: Left midclavicular line at 5th intercostal space.
- o V5: Horizontal to V4 at left anterior axillary line.
- o V6: Horizontal to V5 at left midaxillary line.

In some cases, additional leads may be used:
- Right-sided leads are placed on the right in a mirror image of the left leads, usually to diagnose right ventricular infarction through ST elevation.

## Assessment of heart sounds

Auscultation of heart sounds can help to diagnose different cardiac disorders. Areas to auscultate include the aortic area, pulmonary area, Erb's point, tricuspid area, and the apical area. The normal heart sounds represent closing of the valves.
- The first heart sound (S1) "lub" is closure of the mitral and tricuspid valves (heard at apex/left ventricular area of the heart).
- The second heart sound (S2) "dub" is closure of the aortic and pulmonic valves (heard at the base of the heart). There may be a slight splitting of the S2.

The time between S1 and S1 is systole, and the time between S2 and the next S1 is diastole. Systole and diastole should be silent, although ventricular disease can cause gallops, snaps, or clicks and stenosis of the valves or failure of the valves to close can cause murmurs. Pericarditis may cause a friction rub.

Abnormal heart sounds:

| Abnormal heart sounds | |
|---|---|
| *Gallop rhythms* | *S3* occurs after S2 in children and young adults, but it may indicate heart failure or left ventricular failure in older adults (heard with patient lying on left side). *S4* occurs before S1 and occurs with ventricular hypertrophy, such as from coronary artery disease, hypertension, or aortic valve stenosis. |
| *Opening snap* | An unusual high-pitched sound occurring after S2 with stenosis of mitral valve from rheumatic heart disease. |
| *Ejection click* | A brief high-pitched sound occurring immediately after S1 with stenosis of the aortic valve. |
| *Friction rub* | A harsh, grating sound heard in systole and diastole with pericarditis. |
| *Murmur* | Caused by turbulent blood flow from stenotic or malfunctioning valves, congenital defects, or increased blood flow. Murmurs are characterized by location, timing in the cardiac cycle, intensity (rated from Grade I to Grade VI), pitch (low to high-pitched), quality (rumbling, whistling, blowing) and radiation (to the carotids, axilla, neck, shoulder, or back). |

## Assessing jugular venous pressure

Jugular venous pressure (neck-vein) is used to assess the cardiac output and pressure in the right side of the heart because the pulsations are associated with changes in pressure in the right atrium. This procedure is usually not accurate if pulse rate is >100 bpm. This is a non-invasive estimation of central venous pressure and waveform. Measurement should be done with the internal jugular, if possible; if not, the external jugular may be used.
- Elevate the patient's head to 45° (and to 90° if necessary) with patient's head turned to the right.
- Position the light at an angle to illuminate veins and shadows.
- Measure the height of the jugular vein pulsation above the sternal joint, using a ruler.
  - o Normal height is ≤4 cm above sternal angle.
  - o Increased pressure (>4 cm) indicates increased pressure in right atrium and right heart failure. It may also indicate

*Copyright © Mometrix Media. You have been licensed one copy of this document for personal use only. Any other reproduction or redistribution is strictly prohibited. All rights reserved.*

pericarditis or tricuspid stenosis. Laughing or coughing may trigger the valsalvae response and also cause an increased pulsation.

## Fibrinolytic infusions

Fibrinolytic infusion is indicated for acute myocardial infarction under these conditions:

- Symptoms of MI, <6-12 hours since onset of symptoms.
- ≥1 mm elevation of ST in ≥2 contiguous leads.
- No contraindications and no cardiogenic shock.

Fibrinolytic agents should be administered as soon as possible, within 30 minutes for the best results. All agents convert plasminogen to plasmin, which breaks down fibrin, dissolving clots:

- Streptokinase & anistreplase (1st generation).
- Alteplase or tissue plasminogen activator (tPA) (second generation).
- Reteplase & tenecteplase (3rd generation).

| Contraindications | Relative contraindications |
|---|---|
| Present or recent bleeding or history of severe bleeding. History of brain attack (<2-6 month) or hemorrhagic brain attack. Anticoagulation therapy. Acute uncontrolled hypertension. Aortic dissection or pericarditis. Pregnancy. Intracranial/intraspinal surgery or trauma within 2 months or neoplasm, aneurysm, or arteriovenous malformation (AVM). | Active peptic ulcer. >10 minutes of CPR. >75 years. Advanced renal or hepatic disease. |

## Diuretics

Loop diuretics:
Diuretics increase renal perfusion and filtration, thereby reducing preload and decreasing peripheral and pulmonary edema, hypertension, CHF, diabetes insipidus, and osteoporosis. There are different types of diuretics: loop, thiazide, and potassium sparing.

Loop diuretics inhibit the reabsorption of sodium and chloride (primarily) in the ascending loop of Henle. They also cause increased secretion of other electrolytes, such as calcium, magnesium, and potassium, and this can result in imbalances that cause dysrhythmias. Other side effects include frequent urination, postural hypotension, and increased blood sugar and uric acid levels. Loop diuretics are short-acting, so they are less effective than other diuretics for control of hypertension:

- **Bumetanide** (Bumex®) is given intravenously after surgery to reduce preload or orally to treat heart failure.
- **Ethacrynic acid** (Edecrin®) is given intravenously after surgery to reduce preload.
- **Furosemide** (Lasix®) is used for the control of congestive heart failure as well as renal insufficiency. It is used after surgery to decrease preload and to reduce the inflammatory response caused by cardiopulmonary bypass (post-perfusion syndrome).

Thiazide diuretics:
Thiazide diuretics inhibit the reabsorption of sodium and chloride primarily in the early distal tubules, forcing more sodium and water to be excreted. Thiazide diuretics increase secretion of potassium and bicarbonate, so they are often given with supplementary potassium or in combination with potassium-sparing diuretics. Thiazide diuretics are the first line of drugs for treatment of hypertension. They have a long duration of action (12-72 hours, depending on the drug), so they are able to maintain control of hypertension better than short-acting drugs. They may be given daily or 3-5 days per week.

Copyright © Mometrix Media. You have been licensed one copy of this document for personal use only. Any other reproduction or redistribution is strictly prohibited. All rights reserved.

There are numerous thiazide diuretics, including:

- *Chlorothiazide* (Diuril®).
- *Bendroflumethiazide* (Naturetin®).
- *Chlorthalidone* (Hygroton).
- *Trichlormethiazide* (Naqua®).

Side effects include dizziness, lightheadedness, postural hypotension, headache, blurred vision, and itching, especially during initial treatment. Thiazide diuretics cause sensitivity to sun exposure, so people should be counseled to use sunscreen.

Potassium-sparing diuretics:
Potassium-sparing diuretics inhibit the reabsorption of sodium in the late distal tubule and collecting duct. They are weaker than thiazide or loop diuretics but do not cause a reduction in potassium level; however, if used alone, they may cause an increase in potassium, which can cause weakness, irregular pulse, and cardiac arrest. Because potassium-sparing diuretics are less effective alone, they are often given in a combined form with a thiazide diuretic (usually chlorothiazide), which mitigates the potassium imbalance. Typical side effects include dehydration, blurred vision, nausea, insomnia, and nasal congestion, especially in the first few days of treatment. Drugs in this category include

- *Spironolactone* (Aldactone®) is a synthetic steroid diuretic that increases the secretion of both water and sodium and is used to treat congestive heart failure. It may be given orally or intravenously.
- *Eplerenone* is similar to spironolactone but has fewer side effects, so it may be used with patients who can't tolerate the other drug.

## Digitalis

Digitalis drugs, most commonly administered in the form of digoxin (Lanoxin®), are derived from the foxglove plant and are used to increase myocardial contractility, left ventricular output, and slow conduction through the AV node, as well as to decrease rapid heart rates and promote diuresis. Digoxin does not affect

mortality, but it can increase tolerance to activity and reduce hospitalizations for heart failure. Therapeutic levels (0.5-2.0 ng/mL) should be maintained to avoid digitalis toxicity, which can occur even if digoxin levels are within the therapeutic range, so observation of symptoms is critical. Potassium imbalance may cause toxicity. Evidence of toxicity includes

- Early signs: Increasing fatigue, lethargy, depression, and nausea and vomiting.
- Sudden change in heart rhythm, such as regular or irregular rhythm.
- SA or AV block, new ventricular dysrhythmias, and tachycardia (atrial, junctional, and/or ventricular).

*Treatment* of digitalis toxicity involves discontinuing the medication and monitoring serum levels and symptoms. Digoxin immune FAB (Digibind®) may be used to bind to digoxin and inactivate it, if necessary.

## Vasodilators

Vasodilators may be used for arterial dilation or venous dilation in order to improve cardiac function. These drugs may be used to treat pulmonary hypertension or generalized systemic hypertension. They may be used for those who cannot tolerate ACE inhibitors or angiotensin receptor blockers. Vasodilators may dilate arteries, veins, or both:

- Arterial dilation reduces afterload, improving cardiac output.
- Venous dilation reduces preload, reducing filling pressures.

There are numerous types of vasodilators:

| Smooth muscle relaxants | Decrease peripheral vascular resistance but may cause hypotension and headaches. Sodium nitroprusside (Nipride®) dilates both arteries and veins and is rapid in action; used for reduction of hypertension and afterload reduction for heart failure. Nitroglycerin (Tridil®) primarily dilates veins and is |

Copyright © Mometrix Media. You have been licensed one copy of this document for personal use only. Any other reproduction or redistribution is strictly prohibited. All rights reserved.

| | | | |
|---|---|---|---|
| | given IV to reduce preload for acute heart failure, unstable angina, and acute MI. Nitroglycerin may also be prophylactically after PCIs to prevent vasospasm. Hydralazine (Apresoline®) dilates arteries and is given intermittently to reduce hypertension. | | afterload and preload for heart failure. |
| **Calcium channel blockers** | Primarily arterial vasodilators that may affect the peripheral and/or coronary arteries. Side effects include lethargy, flushing, abdominal and peripheral edema, and indigestion.<br>**Dihydropyridine**, such as nifedipine (Procardia®) (should be avoided in older adults) and nicardipine (Cardene®) are primarily arterial vasodilators affecting both coronary and peripheral arteries; used to treat acute hypertension.<br>**Benzothiazine**, such as diltiazem (Cardizem®) and phenylalkylamine, such as verapamil (Calan®, Isoptin®) dilate primarily coronary arteries and are used for angina and supraventricular tachycardias. | **B-type natriuretic peptide (BNP),** (Nesiritide-Natrecor®) | A new type of vasodilator (non-inotropic), which is a recombinant form of a peptide of the human brain. It decreases filling pressure, vascular resistance, and increases urinary output but may cause hypotension, headache, bradycardia, and nausea. It is used short term for worsening decompensated CHF. |
| | | **Alpha-adrenergic blockers** | Blocks alpha receptors in arteries and veins, causing vasodilation but may cause orthostatic hypotension and edema from fluid retention:<br>**Labetalol (Normodyne®)** is a combination peripheral alpha-blocker and cardiac β-blocker that is used to treat acute hypertension, acute stroke, and acute aortic dissection.<br>**Phentolamine (Regitine®)** is a peripheral arterial dilator that reduces afterload and is used for pheochromocytoma. |
| **Angio-tensin-converting enzyme (ACE) inhibitors** | Limit production of the peripheral vasoconstricting angiotensin, resulting in vasodilation, which can cause a precipitous fall in blood pressure, so use must be carefully monitored. ACE inhibitors are often the first line of drugs to be used for acute hypertension and heart failure; also used to prevent nephropathy in patients with diabetes:<br>**Captopril** (Capoten®) and enalapril (Vasotec®) decrease | **Selec-tive specific dopamine DA-1-receptor agonists** | **Fenoldopam (Corlopam®)** is a peripheral dilator affecting renal and mesenteric arteries that can be used for patients with renal dysfunction or those at risk of renal insufficiency. |

## Glycoprotein IIB/IIIA Inhibitors

Glycoprotein IIB/IIIA Inhibitors are drugs that are used to inhibit platelet binding and prevent clots prior to and following invasive cardiac procedures, such as angioplasty and stent placement. These medications are used in

*Copyright © Mometrix Media. You have been licensed one copy of this document for personal use only. Any other reproduction or redistribution is strictly prohibited. All rights reserved.*

combination with anticoagulant drugs, such as heparin and aspirin for the following:

- *Acute coronary syndromes (ACD)*, such as unstable angina or myocardial infarction.
- *Percutaneous coronary intervention (PCI)*, such as angioplasty and stent placement.

These medications are contraindicated in patients with a low platelet count or active bleeding:

| | |
|---|---|
| **Abciximab (ReoPro®)** | Used with both heparin and aspirin for ACS and PCI; affects platelet binding for 48 hours after administration. |
| **Eptifibatide (Integrilin®)** | Used with both heparin and aspirin for ACS and PCI; affects platelet binding for 6-8 hours after administration. Should not be used for patients with renal problems. |
| **Tirofiban (Aggrastat®)** | Used with heparin for PCI patients, with reduced dosage for those with renal problems; affects platelet blinding for only 4-8 hours after administration |

## Inotropes

Drugs used to increase cardiac output and improve contractibility of the myocardium to treat heart failure are the inotropes. Although intravenous inotropes may increase the risk of death, they may be used when other drugs fail. Oral forms of these drugs are less effective than intravenous. Inotropes include:

| | |
|---|---|
| **β-adren-ergic agonists** | **Dobutamine** improves cardiac output, treats cardiac decompensation, and lowers blood pressure. It helps the body to utilize norepinephrine. Side effects include increases in systolic blood pressure, heart rate, and PVCs (5%); also, hypotension and local reactions. |
| | **Dopamine** improves cardiac output, blood pressure, and the excretion of urine, helping to reduce edema. Side effects include tachycardia or bradycardia, palpitations, BP changes, dyspnea, nausea and vomiting, headache, and gangrene of extremities. |
| **Phosphodiesterase III inhib-itors** | **Milrinone (Primacor®)** increases strength of contractions and cause vasodilation. Side effects include ventricular arrhythmias, hypotension, and headaches. |
| **Digoxin (Lanoxin®)** | Increases contractibility and cardiac output and prevents arrhythmias. |

## Treatment for heart failure

Medications used for heart failure include:

- **ACE inhibitors** *Captopril (Capoten®), enalapril (Vasotec®), and lisinopril (Prinivil®):* Decrease afterload and preload and reverse ventricular remodeling but may cause hypotension initially and are contraindicated with renal insufficiency. Side effects include cough, hyperkalemia, hypotension, angioedema, dizziness, and weakness. Contraindicated with pregnancy and bilateral renal artery stenosis
- **Angiotensin receptor blockers (ARBs)** *Losartan (Cozaar®) and valsartan (Diovan®):* Decrease afterload and preload and reverse ventricular remodeling, causing vasodilation and reducing blood pressure. They are used for those who cannot tolerate ACE inhibitors. Side effects include cough (less common than with ACE inhibitors), hyperkalemia, hypotension, headache, dizziness, metallic taste, and rash.
- **β-blockers** *Metoprolol (Lopressor®), carvedilol (Coreg®) and esmolol (Brevibloc®):* Slow the heart rate, reduce hypertension, prevent dysrhythmias, and reverse ventricular remodeling but should not be used during decompensation; should be

*Copyright © Mometrix Media. You have been licensed one copy of this document for personal use only. Any other reproduction or redistribution is strictly prohibited. All rights reserved.*

monitored carefully for those with airway disease, uncontrolled diabetes, slow irregular pulse, or heart block.
- ***Aldosterone agonist*** *Spironolactone (Aldactone®):* Decreases preload and myocardial hypertrophy and reduces edema and sodium retention but may increase serum potassium.

## Anticoagulants

Anticoagulants are used to prevent thrombo-emboli. All pose risk of bleeding:

| *Aspirin* | Often used prophylactically to prevent clots and poses less danger of bleeding than other drugs. |
|---|---|
| *Warfarin (Coumadin®)* | Blocks utilization of vitamin K. Decreases production of clotting factors and is used orally for those at risk of developing blood clots, such as those with mechanical heart valves, atrial fibrillation, and clotting disorders. |
| *Heparin* | The primary intravenous anticoagulant. It increases the activity of antithrombin III. It is used for patients with MI and those undergoing PCI or other cardiac surgery. |
| *Dalteparin (Fragmin®) & Enoxaparin (Lovenox®)* | Low-molecular weight heparins that increase activity of antithrombin III; used for unstable angina, MI, and cardiac surgery. |
| *Lepirudin (Refludan®) & bivalirudin (Angiomax®)* | Are direct thrombin inhibitors used for unstable angina, PCI, and for prophylaxis and treatment for thrombosis in *heparin-induced thrombo-cytopenia* (allergic response to heparin that causes a platelet count drop [<150,000 per microliter] |

| | usually to 30%-50% of baseline, usually occurring 5-14 days after beginning). |
|---|---|

## Antidysrhythmics

Antidysrhythmics include a number of drugs that act on the conduction system, the ventricles and/or the atria, to control dysrhythmias. There are 4 classes of drugs that are used as well as some that are unclassified:
- Class I:  3 subtypes of sodium channel blockers (quinidine, lidocaine, procainamide).
- Class II: β-receptor blockers (esmolol, propranolol).
- Class III:  Slows repolarization (amiodarone, ibutilide).
- Class IV:  Calcium channel blockers (diltiazem, verapamil).
- Unclassified (Adenosine).

| Antidysrhythmics | |
|---|---|
| *Supra-ventric-ular tachy-cardia* | **Adenosine** affects the conduction system and may cause transient flushing, ↓ BP, and shortness of breath. **Diltiazem (Cardizem®, Tiazac®)** affects the conduction system and may cause bradycardia, AV block, and ↓ BP. **Esmolol (Brevibloc®)** affects the conduction system and may cause ↓ BP, bradycardia, and heart failure. **Propranolol (Inderal®)** affects the conduction system and may cause bradycardia, heart block, and heart failure. **Procainamide** affects the atria and ventricles and may cause ↓ BP and ECG abnormalities (widening of QRS and QT). |

Paroxysmal supraventricular tachycardia: Adenosine. Digoxin (Lanoxin®) affects the conduction system and may cause bradycardia, heart block, nausea and vomiting, and CNS depression. Verapamil (Calan®, Verelan®) affects

*Copyright © Mometrix Media. You have been licensed one copy of this document for personal use only.*
*Any other reproduction or redistribution is strictly prohibited. All rights reserved.*

the conduction system and may cause ↓ BP, bradycardia, and heart failure.

Atrial fibrillation:
Digoxin (Lanoxin®). Diltiazem (Cardizem®, Tiazac®).
Ibutilide (Corvert®) affects the conduction system and rarely has side effects. Amiodarone (Cordarone®) affects the atria and ventricles and may cause ↓ BP, and adverse hepatic effects.

Atrial flutter:
Digoxin (Lanoxin®). Diltiazem (Cardizem®, Tiazac®). Ibutilide (Corvert®). Verapamil (Calan®, Verelan®). Amiodarone (Cordarone®). Procainamide.

Sinus tachycardia:
Esmolol (Brevibloc®).

Premature ventricular contractions:
Lidocaine affects the ventricles and may cause CNS toxicity with nausea and vomiting.
Procainamide

Ventricular tachycardia:
Lidocaine. Amiodarone (Cardizem®, Tiazac®).
Procainamide

Ventricular fibrillation:
Lidocaine

## Pulmonary

### Acute lung injury

Acute lung injury (ALI) comprises a syndrome of respiratory distress culminating in *acute respiratory distress syndrome (ARDS).* ALI/ARDS is characterized by respiratory distress within 72 hours of surgery or a serious injury (including smoke inhalation, near-drowning, or head injury causing pulmonary edema) to a person with otherwise normal lungs and heart. ARDS is defined as damage to the vascular endothelium from an increase in the permeability of the alveolar-capillary membrane. This occurs when damage to the lung results in

toxic substances (such as gastric fluids, bacteria, chemicals, or toxins [emitted by neutrophils as part of the inflammatory-mediated response]) that reduce surfactant, causing pulmonary edema (as the alveoli fill with blood and protein-rich fluid) and collapse. Atelectasis with hyperinflation and areas of normal tissue occur as the lungs "stiffen." The fluid in the alveoli becomes a medium for infection. Because there is neither adequate ventilation nor perfusion, the result is increasing hypoxemia and tachypnea as the body tries to compensate to maintain a normal partial pressure of carbon dioxide ($PaCO_2$). Untreated, the condition results in respiratory failure, multi-organ failure, and death.

Symptoms:
Patients presenting with **acute lung injury (ALI)/acute respiratory distress syndrome (ARDS)** may initially present with only mild tachypnea, but more serious *symptoms* develop as respiratory function becomes more compromised:

- Crackling rales or wheezing may be heard throughout the lungs.
- Decrease in pulmonary compliance (lung volume), referred to as "baby lung," results in increasing tachypnea with expiratory grunting.
- Cyanosis may develop with characteristic blue discoloration of lips and skin mottling.
- Hypotension and tachycardia may occur.
- Symptoms associated with volume overload are missing (3rd heart sound or jugular venous distention).
- Respiratory alkalosis is often an early sign but is replaced as the disease progresses with hypercarbia and respiratory acidosis.
- X-ray studies may be normal at first but then show diffuse infiltrates in both lungs, but the heart and vessels appear normal.

Management:
The management of acute lung injury/acute respiratory distress syndrome (ALI/ARDS) involves providing adequate gas exchange and preventing further damage to the lung from forced ventilation. *Treatment* includes:

*Copyright © Mometrix Media. You have been licensed one copy of this document for personal use only.*
*Any other reproduction or redistribution is strictly prohibited. All rights reserved.*

- Oxygen therapy by nasal prongs/cannula or mask may be sufficient in mild cases to maintain oxygen saturation above 90%. Oxygen should be administered at 100% because of the mismatch between ventilation (V) and perfusion (Q), which can result in hypoxia on position change.
- Endotracheal intubation may be needed if oxygen saturation falls or carbon dioxide levels rise.
- Mechanical ventilation with lower tidal volumes or high-frequency oscillatory ventilation may be needed to maintain oxygen saturation >90%.
- Inhaled nitric oxide may be prescribed for pulmonary hypertension.
- Prophylactic antibiotics are not indicated.
- Steroids may increase survival rates if given later in treatment if ARDS has not resolved within a week.

Placing patient in prone position 18-24 hours/day with chest and pelvis supported and abdomen unsupported allows the diaphragm to move posteriorly, increasing functional residual capacity (FRC).

## Aspiration pneumonitis

There are a number of risk factors that can lead to aspiration pneumonitis/pneumonia:
- Altered level of consciousness related to illness or sedation.
- Diseases (Alzheimer's, Parkinson's)
- Depression of gag, swallowing reflex.
- Intubation or feeding tubes.
- Ileus or gastric distention.
- Gastrointestinal disorders, such as gastroesophageal reflux disorders (GERD).

*Diagnosis* is based on clinical findings, arterial blood gas (ABGs) showing hypoxemia, infiltrates observed on x-ray, and ↑ WBC if infection is present. *Symptoms* are similar to other pneumonias, depending upon the site of inflammation: cough often with copious sputum, dyspnea, respiratory distress, cyanosis, tachycardia, and hypotension.

*Treatment* includes:
- Suctioning as needed to clear upper airway.
- Supplemental oxygen.
- Antibiotic therapy as indicated after 48 hours if symptoms are not resolving.
- Symptomatic respiratory support.

## Foreign body aspiration

Foreign body aspiration can cause obstruction of the pharynx, larynx or trachea, leading to acute dyspnea or asphyxiation, and the object may be drawn distally into the bronchial tree. With adults, most foreign bodies migrate more readily down the right bronchus. Infants and children, especially those weak or ill, are prone to aspiration of foreign substances (food, powder, secretions) or objects (dry nuts, candy, popcorn, toys). Sometimes the object causes swelling, ulceration, and general inflammation that hamper removal. *Symptoms* include:
- ***Initial***: Severe coughing, gagging, sternal retraction, wheezing. Objects in the larynx may cause inability to breathe or speak and lead to respiratory arrest. Objects in the bronchus cause cough, dyspnea, and wheezing.
- ***Delayed***: Hours, days, or weeks later, an undetected aspirant may cause an infection distal to the aspirated material. Symptoms depend on the area and extent of the infection.

*Treatment* includes:
- Heimlich maneuver (first responder) if no respirations.
- Removal with laryngoscopy or bronchoscopy (rigid is often better than flexible).
- Antibiotic therapy for secondary infection.
- Surgical bronchotomy (rare).
- Symptomatic support.

## Positive pressure ventilators

Positive pressure ventilators assist respiration by applying pressure directly to the airway, inflating the lungs, forcing expansion of the alveoli, and facilitating gas exchange. Generally,

*Copyright © Mometrix Media. You have been licensed one copy of this document for personal use only. Any other reproduction or redistribution is strictly prohibited. All rights reserved.*

endotracheal intubation or tracheostomy is necessary to maintain positive pressure ventilation for extended periods. There are 3 basic kinds of positive pressure ventilators:

- *Pressure cycled:* This type of ventilation is usually used for short-term treatment in adolescents or adults. The IPPB machine is the most common type. This delivers a flow of air to a preset pressure and then cycles off. Airway resistance or changes in compliance can affect the volume of air and may compromise ventilation.
- *Time cycled:* This type of ventilation regulates the volume of air the patient receives by controlling the length of inspiration and the flow rate.
- *Volume cycled:* This type of ventilation provides a preset flow of pressurized air during inspiration and then cycles off, allowing passive expiration and providing a fairly consistent volume of air.

## Non-invasive positive pressure ventilators

Non-invasive positive pressure ventilators provide air through a tight-fitting nasal or facemask, usually pressure cycled, avoiding the need for intubation and reducing the danger of hospital-acquired infection and mortality rates. It can be used for acute respiratory failure and pulmonary edema. There are 2 types of non-invasive positive pressure ventilators:

- *CPAP (Continuous positive airway pressure)* provides a steady stream of pressurized air throughout both inspiration and expiration. CPAP improves breathing by decreasing preload and afterload for patients with congestive heart failure. It reduces the effort required for breathing and improves compliance of the lung.
- *Bi-PAP (Bi-level positive airway pressure)* provides a steady stream of pressurized air as CPAP, but it senses inspiratory effort and increases pressure during inspiration. Bi-PAP pressures for inspiration and expiration can be set independently. Machines can be programmed with a backup rate to ensure a set number of respirations per minute.

## High frequency jet ventilation

High frequency jet ventilation (HFJV) (Life Pulse®) directs a high velocity stream of air into the lungs in a long spiraling spike that forces carbon dioxide against the walls, penetrating dead space and providing gas exchange by using small tidal volumes of 1-3 ml/kg, much smaller than with conventional mechanical ventilation. Because the jet stream technology is effective for short distances, the valve and pressure transducer must be placed by the person's head. Inhalation is controlled while expiration is passive, but the rate of respiration is up to 11 per second ("panting" respirations). HFJV may be used in conjunction with low-pressure conventional ventilation to increase flow to alveoli. HFJV reduces barotrauma because of the low tidal volume and low pressure. HFJV is used for numerous conditions, including evolving chronic lung disease, pulmonary interstitial emphysema, bronchopulmonary dysplasia, and hypoxemic respiratory failure. It reduces mean airway pressure (MAP) and the oxygenation index. Treatment with HFJV may reduce the need for extra corporeal membrane oxygenation (ECMO).

## High frequency oscillatory ventilation

High frequency oscillatory ventilation (HFOV) provides pressurized ventilation with tidal volumes approximately equal to dead space at about 150 breaths per minutes (bpm). Pressure is usually higher with HFOV than HFJV in order to maintain expansion of the alveoli and to keep the airway open during gas exchange. Oxygenation is regulated separately. HFOV has both an active inspiration and expiration, so the respiratory cycle is completely controlled. HFOV reduces pulmonary vascular resistance and improves ventilation-perfusion matching and oxygenation without injuring the lung, reducing the risk of barotrauma. HFOV is used for respiratory distress syndrome, persistent pulmonary hypertension, more commonly for infants and children. However, there is increasing interest in using HFOV with adults because of the smaller tidal volume that

*Copyright © Mometrix Media. You have been licensed one copy of this document for personal use only. Any other reproduction or redistribution is strictly prohibited. All rights reserved.*

prevents overinflation of the lungs and atelectasis of those with ARDS. Use of HFOV decreases barotrauma associated with ventilation.

## Ventilation-induced lung injury

Ventilation-induced lung injury (VILI) is damage caused by mechanical ventilation. It is common in acute respiratory distress syndrome (ARDS) but can affect any ventilation patient. VILI comprises 4 interrelated elements:

- **Barotrauma**: Damage to the lung caused by excessive pressure.
- **Volutrauma**: Alveolar damage related to high tidal volume ventilation.
- **Atelectotrauma**: Injury caused by repetitive forced opening and closing of alveoli.
- **Biotrauma**: Inflammatory response.

In VILI, essentially, the increased pressure and tidal volume over-distends the alveoli which rupture, and air moves into the interstitial tissue resulting in pulmonary interstitial emphysema. With continued ventilation, the air in the interstitium moves into the subcutaneous tissue and may result in pneumopericardium and pneumomediastinum. Alternatively, rupture of the pleural sac can cause tension pneumothorax and mediastinal shift, which can lead to respiratory failure and cardiac arrest. VILI has caused a change in ventilation procedures so that lower tidal volumes and pressures are used as well as newer forms of ventilation, i.e., HFJV and HFOV that are preferred to mechanical ventilation for many patients.

## Chronic ventilatory failure

Chronic ventilatory failure occurs when alveolar ventilation fails to increase in response to increasing levels of carbon dioxide, usually associated with chronic pulmonary diseases, such as asthma and COPD, drug overdoses, or diseases that impair respiratory effort, such as Guillain-Barré and myasthenia gravis. Normally, the ventilatory system is able to maintain $PCO_2$ and pH levels within narrow limits, even though $PO_2$ levels may be more variable, but with ventilatory failure, the body is not able to compensate for the resultant hypercapnia, and pH falls, resulting in respiratory acidosis. *Symptoms* include increasing dyspnea with tachypnea, gasping respirations, and use of accessory muscles. Patients may become confused as hypercapnia causes increased intracranial pressure. If pH is <7.2 (neutral pH = 7.35 to 7.45), cardiac arrhythmias, hyperkalemia, and hypotension can occur as pulmonary arteries constrict and the peripheral vascular system dilates. Diagnosis is per symptoms, ABGs consistent with respiratory acidosis ($PCO_2$ >50 mm Hg and pH <7.35), pulse oximetry, and chest x-ray. *Treatment* can include non-invasive positive pressure ventilation (PPV), endotracheal mechanical ventilation, corticosteroids, and bronchodilators.

## Ventilator management

There are many types of ventilators now in use, and the specific directions for use of each type must be followed carefully, but there are general principles that apply to all ventilator management. The following should be monitored:

- **Type of ventilation:** volume-cycled, pressure-cycled, negative-pressure, HFJV, HFOV, CPAP, Bi-PAP.
- **Control mode:** controlled ventilation, assisted ventilation, synchronized intermittent mandatory (allows spontaneous breaths between ventilator controlled inhalation/exhalation), positive-end expiratory pressure (positive pressure at end of expiration [PEEP]), CPAP, Bi-PAP.
- **Tidal volume** $(T_v)$ range should be set in relation to respiratory rate.
- **Inspiratory-expiratory ratio** (I:E) usually ranges from 1:2-1:5, but may vary.
- **Respiratory rate** will depend upon $T_v$ and $PaCO_2$ target.
- **Fraction of inspired oxygen** ($FiO_2$, percentage of oxygen in the inspired air), usually ranging from 21%-100%, usually maintained <40% to avoid toxicity.
- **Sensitivity** determines the effort needed to trigger inspiration.

*Copyright © Mometrix Media. You have been licensed one copy of this document for personal use only. Any other reproduction or redistribution is strictly prohibited. All rights reserved.*

- **Pressure** controls the pressure exerted in delivering $T_v$.
- **Rate of flow** controls the L/min speed of $T_v$.

Facemask:
Ensuring that a facemask fits correctly and is the correct type is important for adequate ventilation, oxygenation, and prevention of aspiration. Difficulties in the management of facemask ventilation relate to risk factors: >55 years, obesity, beard, edentulous, and history of snoring. In some cases, if dentures are adhered well, they may be left in place during induction. The facemask is applied by lifting the mandible (jaw thrust) to the mask and avoiding pressure on soft tissue. Oral or nasal airways may be used, ensuring that the distal end is at the angle of the mandible. There are a number of steps to prevent mask airway leaks:

- Increasing or decreasing the amount of air to the mask to allow better seal.
- Securing the mask with both hands while another person ventilates.
- Accommodating a large nose by using the mask upside down.
- Utilizing a laryngeal mask airway if excessive beard prevents seal.

Nasal cannula:
A nasal cannula can be used to deliver supplemental oxygen to a patient, but it is only useful for flow rates ≤ 6 L/min because higher rates cause drying of the nasal passages. As it is not an airtight system, some ambient air is breathed in as well, so the oxygen concentration will range from about 24%-44%. The nasal cannula does not allow for control of respiratory rate, so the patient must be able to breathe independently.

Non-rebreather mask:
A non-rebreather mask can be used to deliver higher concentrations (60%-90%) of oxygen to those patients who are able to breathe independently. The mask fits over the nose and mouth and is secured by an elastic strap. A 1.5 L reservoir bag is attached and connects to an oxygen source. The bag is inflated to about 1 liter at a rate of 8-15 L/min before the mask is applied, as the patient breathes from this reservoir. A one-way exhalation valve prevents most exhaled air from being rebreathed.

**Arterial blood gases**

Arterial blood gases are monitored to assess effectiveness of oxygenation, ventilation, and acid-base status and to determine oxygen flow rates. The partial pressure of a gas is that exerted by each gas in a mixture of gases, proportional to its concentration, based on total atmospheric pressure of 760 mm Hg at sea level. Normal values include:

- Acidity/alkalinity (pH): 7.35-7.45.
- Partial pressure of carbon dioxide ($PaCO_2$): 35-45 mm Hg.
- Partial pressure of oxygen ($PaO_2$): ≥80 mg Hg.
- Bicarbonate concentration ($HCO_3$): 22-26 mEq/L.
- Oxygen saturation ($SaO_2$): ≥95%.

The relationship between these elements, particularly the $PaCO_2$ and the $PaO_2$ indicates respiratory status. For example, $PaCO_2$ >55 and the $PaO_2$ <60 in a patient previously in good health indicates respiratory failure. There are many issues to consider. Ventilator management may require a higher $PaCO2$ to prevent barotrauma and a lower $PaO_2$ to reduce oxygen toxicity.

**Respiratory acidosis**

Respiratory acidosis is precipitated by inadequate ventilation of alveoli, interfering with gaseous exchange so that carbon dioxide increases and oxygen decreases, causing excess carbonic acid ($H_2CO_3$) levels. The body maintains a normal pH by balancing bicarbonate (renal) with $PaCO_2$ (pulmonary) in a 20:1 ratio. If the pH alters, the system (renal or pulmonary) that is not causing the problem compensates. Respiratory acidosis is common in acute respiratory disorders, such as pulmonary edema, pneumothorax, sleep apnea syndrome, atelectasis, aspiration of foreign objects, severe pneumonia, ARDS, administration of oxygen to

Copyright © Mometrix Media. You have been licensed one copy of this document for personal use only. Any other reproduction or redistribution is strictly prohibited. All rights reserved.

treat chronic hypercapnia, or mechanical ventilation. Diseases with respiratory muscle impairment may also cause respiratory acidosis, such as muscular dystrophy, severe Guillain-Barré, and myasthenia gravis. Respiratory acidosis may be acute or chronic:

- **Acute**: $\uparrow PaCO_2$ with $\downarrow$ pH caused by sudden decrease in ventilation.
- **Chronic**: $\uparrow PaCO_2$ with normal pH and serum bicarbonate ($HCO_3$) >30 mm Hg with renal compensation.

Normal ABG values in respiratory acidosis:
- pH <7.35.
- $PaCO_2$ >42 mm Hg.
- $\uparrow H_2CO_3$.

Symptoms and treatment:
Symptoms of respiratory acidosis may vary considerably. *Symptoms* of acute respiratory acidosis may include:

- $\uparrow$ Heart rate, hypertension, ventricular fibrillation.
- Tachypnea.
- Confusion and pressure in head related to cerebrovascular vasodilation, especially if $PaCO_2$ >60 mm Hg, $\uparrow$ intracranial pressure with papilledema.
- Hyperkalemia.

Symptoms may be more subtle with chronic respiratory acidosis because of the compensatory mechanisms. This is especially true of patients with COPD who gradually increase levels of $CO_2$; they may not develop symptoms of hypercapnia because the kidneys have time to compensate. If the $PaCO_2$ remains >50 mm Hg for long periods, the respiratory center becomes increasingly insensitive to CO2 as a respiratory stimulus, replaced by hypoxemia, so supplemental oxygen administration should be monitored carefully to ensure that respirations are not depressed.
*Treatment* includes:

- Improving ventilation.
- Medications as indicated (depending on cause): bronchodilators, anticoagulation therapy, diuretics, and antibiotics.

- Pulmonary hygiene.
- Mechanical ventilation may be used with care.

**Respiratory alkalosis**

Respiratory alkalosis results from hyperventilation, during which extra $CO_2$ is excreted, causing a decrease in carbonic acid ($H_2CO_3$) concentration in the plasma. Respiratory alkalosis may be acute or chronic. Acute respiratory alkalosis is precipitated by anxiety attacks, hypoxemia, salicylate intoxication, bacteremia (Gram-negative), and incorrect ventilator settings. Chronic respiratory alkalosis may result from chronic hepatic insufficiency, cerebral tumors, and chronic hypocapnia. Respiratory alkalosis is characterized by:
$\downarrow PaCO_2$ and $\uparrow$ pH. Normal or decreased serum bicarbonate ($HCO_3$) as kidneys conserve hydrogen and excrete $HCO_3$.

*Symptoms* include:
Vasoconstriction with $\downarrow$ cerebral blood flow resulting in lightheadedness, alterations in mentation, and/or unconsciousness. Numbness and tingling, tinnitus. Tachycardia and dysrhythmias.
*Treatment* includes identifying and treating underlying cause. If respiratory alkalosis is related to anxiety, breathing in a paper bag may increase $CO_2$ level. Some people may require sedation. Common ABG values in respiratory alkalosis:

- pH >7.45.
- $PaCO_2$ <38 mm Hg.
- $H_2CO_3$.

**COPD**

Functional dyspnea, body mass index (BMI), and spirometry are used to assess the stages of COPD. The spirometry measures used are the ratio of forced expiratory volume in the 1st second of expiration ($FEV_1$) after full inhalation to total forced vital capacity (FVC). Normal lung function decreases after age 35; so normal

*Copyright © Mometrix Media. You have been licensed one copy of this document for personal use only. Any other reproduction or redistribution is strictly prohibited. All rights reserved.*

values are adjusted for height, weight, sex, and age:

- **Stage 1** (mild): Minimal dyspnea with/without cough and sputum. $FEV_1$ is ≥80% of predicted rate and $FEV_1$:FVC = <70%.
- **Stage 2** (moderate): Moderate to severe chronic exertional dyspnea with/without cough and sputum. $FEV_1$ is 50%-80% of predicted rate and $FEV_1$:FVC = <70%.
- **Stage 3** (severe): As in stage 2 but repeated episodes with increased exertional dyspnea and the condition impacting the patient's quality of life. $FEV_1$ is 30%-50% of predicted rate and $FEV_1$:FVC = <70%.
- **Stage 4** (very severe): Severe dyspnea and life-threatening episodes that severely impact the quality of life. $FEV_1$ is 30% of predicted rate or <50% with chronic respiratory failure and $FEV_1$:FVC = <70%.

Acute exacerbation:
Acute exacerbations of chronic obstructive pulmonary disease (COPD) usually require hospitalized treatment. COPD is not reversible, so management aims at slowing progression, relieving symptoms, and improving quality of life. COPD may be emphysema predominant (pink puffer) or bronchitis predominant (blue bloater). Treatment includes:

- **Bronchodilators**, such as short-acting anticholinergic ipratropium bromide and β-2 agonists (albuterol [Ventolin®]) for bronchospasm and airway obstruction. These should be discontinued if they do not relieve symptoms. Long-acting β-2 agonists (such as formoterol and salmeterol) are often more effective.
- **Corticosteroids**, both inhaled (Pulmicort®, Vanceril®) and oral (prednisone) may improve symptoms.
- **Theophylline** is usually not initiated with acute exacerbations unless there is no response to bronchodilators or corticosteroids.
- **Supplemental oxygen therapy** is given to relieve hypoxemia.

- **Antibiotics** (macrolides, fluoroquinolones, or amoxicillin-clavulanate) are usually given, especially if there is a change in the quality of sputum.
- **Chest physiotherapy** may be indicated for some patients with excessive secretions.

**Pneumothorax**

Pneumothorax is a leak between the lung tissue and the chest wall, so extraneous air is in the pleural space. Types include:

- **Spontaneous/Simple pneumothorax** is a breach of the parietal or visceral pleura occurring when an air-filled bleb on the lung surface ruptures or from a bronchopleural fistula without connection to outside air.
- **Traumatic pneumothorax** is a lacerating wound of the chest wall, such as a gunshot or knife wound. It can also result from invasive procedures, such as thoracentesis or lung biopsies, or from barotrauma related to ventilation or chest surgery. Open pneumothorax occurs when air passes in and out, causing the lung to collapse, causing a sucking sound, and paradoxical movement of the chest wall with respirations.
- **Tension pneumothorax** is similar to traumatic open pneumothorax; however, the air can enter the pleural sac but can't be expelled, causing a pronounced mediastinal shift to the unaffected side with severe compromise of cardiac and respiratory function.

Symptoms, diagnosis, and treatment:
Pneumothorax occurs when there is a leak of air into the pleural space, resulting in complete or partial collapse of a lung:

| Symptoms | Vary widely, depending on the cause and degree of the pneumothorax and whether or not there is underlying disease: Acute pleuritic pain (95%), usually on the affected side. Decreased breath sounds. Tension pneumothorax: tracheal deviation and hemodynamic compromise. |
|---|---|

Copyright © Mometrix Media. You have been licensed one copy of this document for personal use only. Any other reproduction or redistribution is strictly prohibited. All rights reserved.

| | |
|---|---|
| **Diagnosis** | Clinical findings. Radiograph: 6-foot upright posterior-anterior. Ultrasound may detect traumatic pneumothorax. |
| **Treatment** | Chest-tube thoracostomy with underwater seal drainage is the most common treatment for all types of pneumothorax. Tension pneumothorax: Immediate needle decompression and chest tube thoracostomy. Small pneumothorax: Oxygen administration (3-4 L/min) and observation for 3-6 hours. If no increase is shown on repeat x-ray, patient may be discharged with another x-ray in 24-48 hours. Primary spontaneous pneumothorax: catheter aspiration or chest tube thoracostomy. |

## Thoracic hemothorax

Hemothorax occurs with bleeding into the pleural space, usually from major vascular injury, such as tears in intercostal vessels, lacerations of great vessels, or trauma to lung parenchyma. A small bleed may be self-limiting and seal, but a tear in a large vessel can result in massive bleeding, followed quickly by hypovolemic shock. The pressure from the blood may result in inability of the lung to ventilate and a mediastinal shift. Often a hemothorax occurs with a pneumothorax, especially in severe chest trauma. Further symptoms include severe respiratory distress, decreased breath sounds, and dullness on auscultation. Treatment includes placement of a chest tube to drain the hemothorax, but with large volumes, the pressure may be preventing exsanguination, which can occur abruptly as the blood drains and pressure is reduced, so a large bore intravenous line should be in place and typed and cross-matched blood immediately available

prior to chest tube insertion. Autotransfusion may be used.

## Thoracentesis

A thoracentesis (aspiration of fluid or air from pleural space) is done to make a diagnosis, relieve pressure on the lung caused by pleural effusion, or instill medications. A chest x-ray is done prior to the procedure. A sedative may be given. The patient is in sitting position, leaning onto a padded bedside stand, straddling a chair with head supported on the back of the chair, or lying on the opposite side with the head of the bed elevated 30º-45° to ensure that fluid remains at the base. The patient should avoid coughing or moving during the procedure. The chest x-ray or ultrasound determines needle placement. After a local anesthetic is administered, a needle (with an attached 20-ml syringe and 3-way stopcock with tubing and a receptacle) is advanced intercostally into the pleural space. Fluid is drained, collected, examined, and measured. The needle is removed and a pressure dressing applied. A chest x-ray is done to ensure there is no pneumothorax. The patient is monitored for cough, dyspnea, and hypoxemia.

## Chest tubes

Chest tubes with a closed drainage system are usually left in place after thoracic surgery or pneumothorax treatment to drain air or fluid:

- *Water seal (wet suction):* 3-chambered system with 1 chamber for collection, the middle for water seal, and the 3rd for wet suction control. Sterile fluid must be instilled into the middle and suction chambers. Contains both positive and negative pressure release valves and bubbles intermittently if functioning properly. Must be in an upright position.
- *Water seal (dry suction):* Similar 3-chambered system, but sterile fluid must be instilled to 2-cm level in water seal chamber only. A regulator controls suction, and an indicator shows if the suction pressure is

- 45 -

*Copyright © Mometrix Media. You have been licensed one copy of this document for personal use only. Any other reproduction or redistribution is strictly prohibited. All rights reserved.*

correct. Has positive and negative release values. Must be in an upright position.

- **Dry suction (one-way valve):** 2-chambered system with a mechanical valve that allows air to leave the chest but not enter. Has a collection chamber and a dry suction control chamber. Requires no fluid instillation and need not be in an upright position, which makes it useful for ambulatory patients.

## Pulmonary trauma/disease

The diagnostic procedures and tools used during assessment of pulmonary and thoracic trauma/disease will vary according to the type and degree of injury/disease, but may include:

- **Thorough physical examination** including cardiac and pulmonary status, assessing for any abnormalities.
- **Electrocardiogram** assessment for cardiac arrhythmias.
- **Chest x-ray** should be done for all patients with injuries to check for fractures, pneumothorax, major injuries, and placement of intubation tubes. X-rays can be taken quickly with portable equipment, so they can be completed quickly during the initial assessment.
- **Computerized tomography** may be indicated after initial assessment, especially if there is a possibility of damage to the parenchyma of the lungs.
- **Oximetry and atrial blood gases** as indicated.
- **12-lead electrocardiogram** may be needed for more careful observation if there are arrhythmias.
- **Echocardiogram** should be done if there is apparent cardiac damage.

## Pulmonary pharmacology

There are a wide range of agents used for pulmonary pharmacology, depending upon the type and degree of pulmonary disease. Agents include:

- **Opioid analgesics:** Use to provide both pain relief and sedation for those on mechanical ventilation to reduce sympathetic response. Medications may include fentanyl (Sublimaze®) or morphine sulfate (MS Contin®).
- **Neuromuscular blockers:** Used for induced paralysis of patients who have not responded adequately to sedation, especially for intubation and mechanical ventilation. Medications may include pancuronium (Pavulon®) and vecuronium (Norcuron®). However, there is controversy about the use because induced paralysis has been linked to increased mortality rates, sensory hearing loss (pancuronium), atelectasis, and ventilation-perfusion mismatch.
- **Human B-type natriuretic peptides:** Used to reduce pulmonary capillary wedge pressure. Medications include nesiritide (Natrecor®).
- **Vasopressors/Inotropes:** Used to increase cardiac output. Dopamine (Intropin®) increases renal output and blood pressure. Dobutamine (Dobutrex®) increases cardiac contractibility and blood pressure.
- **Surfactants:** Reduces surface tension to prevent collapse of alveoli. Beractant (Survanta®) is derived from bovine lung tissue, and calfactant (Infasurf®) is derived from calf lung tissue. They are administered as inhalants.
- **Alkalinizers:** Used to treat metabolic acidosis and ↓ pulmonary vascular resistance by achieving an alkaline pH. Medications include sodium bicarbonate and tromethamine (THAM).
- **Pulmonary vasodilator (inhaled nitrous oxide):** Used to relax the vascular muscles and produce pulmonary vasodilation. Some studies show it reduces the need for extracorporeal membrane oxygenation (ECMO), although this is not supported by other studies.
- **Methylxanthines:** Used to stimulate muscle contractions of the chest and stimulate respirations. Medications include aminophylline (Aminophylline®), caffeine citrate (Cafcit®), and doxapram (Dopram®).

*Copyright © Mometrix Media. You have been licensed one copy of this document for personal use only. Any other reproduction or redistribution is strictly prohibited. All rights reserved.*

- **Diuretics:** Used to reduce pulmonary edema. Medications include loop diuretics such as furosemide (Lasix®) and metolazone (Mykrox®).
- **Nitrates:** Used for vasodilation to reduce preload and afterload in order to reduce myocardial need for oxygen. Medications include nitroglycerin (Nitro-Bid®) and nitroprusside sodium (Nitropress®).
- **Antibiotics:** Used for treatment of respiratory infections, including pneumonia. Medications are used according to the pathogenic agent and may include macrolides, such as azithromycin (Zithromax®), erythromycin (E-Mycin®).
- **Antimycobacterials:** Used for treatment of TB and other mycobacterial diseases. Medications include isoniazid (Laniazid®, Nydrazid®), ethambutol (Myambutol®), rifampin (Rifadin®), streptomycin sulfate, and pyrazinamide.
- **Antivirals:** Used to inhibit replication of virus early in a viral infection. Effectiveness decreases as time passes because the replication process has already begun. Medications include ribavirin (Virazole®) and zanamivir (Relenza®).

## Acute pulmonary embolism

Acute pulmonary embolism occurs when a pulmonary artery or arteriole is blocked by a blood clot originating in the venous system or the right heart. While most pulmonary emboli are from thrombus formation, other causes may be air, fat, or septic embolus (from bacterial invasion of a thrombus). Common originating sites for thrombus formation are the deep veins in the legs, the pelvic veins, and the right atrium. Causes include stasis related to damage to endothelial wall and changes in blood coagulation factors. Atrial fibrillation poses a serious risk because blood pools in the right atrium, forming clots that travel directly through the right ventricle to the lungs. The obstruction of the artery/arteriole causes an increase in alveolar dead space in which there is ventilation but impairment of gas exchange because of the ventilation/perfusion mismatching or intrapulmonary shunting. This results in hypoxia, hypercapnia, and the release of mediators that cause bronchoconstriction. If more than 50% of the vascular bed becomes excluded, pulmonary hypertension occurs.

Symptoms and diagnosis:
Clinical manifestations of acute pulmonary embolism (PE) vary according to the size of the embolus and the area of occlusion. Common presenting *symptoms* include:
- Dyspnea with tachypnea, cough (sometimes with hemoptysis), rales, chest pain.
- Tachycardia, hemodynamic instability.
- Anxiety, restlessness, and fever.

- A clinical diagnosis is supported by *diagnostic* tests, which may include
- ABG analysis may show hypoxemia ($\downarrow$ PaO2), hypocarbia ($\downarrow$ PaCO2) and respiratory alkalosis ($\uparrow$ pH).
- D-dimer (will show elevation with PE).
- ECG may show sinus tachycardia or other abnormalities.
- Echocardiogram can show emboli in the central arteries and can assess the hemodynamic status of the right side of the heart.
- Chest x-ray is of minimal value.
- Spiral CT may provide definitive diagnosis.
- V/Q scintigraphy can confirm diagnosis.
- Pulmonary angiograms also can confirm diagnosis.

Medical management:
Medical management of pulmonary embolism starts with preventive measures for those at risk, including leg exercises, elastic compression stockings, and anticoagulation therapy (Coumadin®). Most pulmonary emboli present as medical emergencies, so the immediate task is to stabilize the patient. Medical management may include:
- *Oxygen* to relieve hypoxemia.
- *Intravenous* infusions.
- *Dobutamine* (Dobutrex®) or dopamine (Intropin®) to relieve hypotension.
- *Cardiac monitoring* for dysrhythmias.

*Copyright © Mometrix Media. You have been licensed one copy of this document for personal use only. Any other reproduction or redistribution is strictly prohibited. All rights reserved.*

- *Medications* as indicated: digitalis glycosides, diuretic, and antiarrhythmics.
- *Intubation and mechanical ventilation* may be required.
- *Analgesia* (such as morphine sulfate) or sedation to relieve anxiety.
- *Anticoagulants* to prevent recurrence (although it will not dissolve clots already present), including heparin and warfarin (Coumadin®).
- *Placement of percutaneous venous filter* (Greenfield) in the inferior vena cava to prevent further emboli from entering the lungs may be done if anticoagulation therapy is contraindicated.
- *Thrombolytic therapy*, recombinant tissue-type plasminogen activator (rt-PA) or streptokinase, for those severely compromised, but these treatments have limited success and pose the danger of bleeding.

## Pulmonary hypertension

Pulmonary arterial hypertension (PAH) may involve multiple processes. Usually the pulmonary vasculature adjusts easily to accommodate blood volume from the right ventricle. If there is increased blood flow, the low resistance causes vasodilation and *vice versa*. However, sometimes the pulmonary vascular bed is damaged or obstructed, and this can impair the ability to handle changing volumes of blood. In that case, an increase in flow will increase the pulmonary arterial pressure, increasing pulmonary vascular resistance (PVR). This, in turn, increases pressure on the right ventricle (RV) with increased RV workload and eventual RV hypertrophy, as well as displacement of the intraventricular septum and tricuspid regurgitation. Over time, this leads to right heart failure and death. Pulmonary hypertension is usually diagnosed by right-sided heart catheterization and is indicated by systolic pulmonary artery pressure >30 mm Hg and mean pulmonary artery pressure >25 mm Hg. Non-invasive testing may be done using an echocardiogram to look for cardiac changes.

Classifications:
Pulmonary hypertension or pulmonary arterial hypertension (PAH) is a progressive disease of the pulmonary arteries that can severely compromise cardiovascular patients. PAH may be classified as primary (idiopathic) or secondary:
- ***Primary (idiopathic) PAH*** may result from changes in immune responses, pulmonary emboli, sickle cell disease, collagen diseases, Raynaud's, and the use of contraceptives. The cause may be unknown or genetic.
- ***Secondary PAH*** may result from pulmonary vasoconstriction brought on by hypoxemia related to COPD, sleep-disordered breathing, kyphoscoliosis, obesity, smoke inhalation, altitude sickness, interstitial pneumonia, and neuromuscular disorders. It may also be caused by a decrease in the pulmonary vascular bed of 50%-75%, which may result from pulmonary emboli, vasculitis, tumor emboli, and interstitial lung disease, such as sarcoidosis. Primary cardiac disease, such as congenital defects in infants, and acquired disorders, such as rheumatic valve disease, mitral stenosis, and left ventricular failure may also contribute to PAH.

Treatment options:
Medical treatment for pulmonary arterial hypertension (PAH) aims to identify and treat any underlying cardiac or pulmonary disease, control symptoms, and prevent complications:
- *Oxygen therapy* may be needed, especially supplemental oxygen during exercise.
- *Calcium channel blockers* may provide vasodilation for some patients.
- *Pulmonary vascular dilators,* such as IV epoprostenol (Flolan®) and subcutaneous treprostinil sodium (Remodulin® and oral bosentan [Tracleer®]) help to control symptoms and prolong life.
- *Anticoagulation*, such as warfarin (Coumadin®) is an important part of therapy because of recurrent pulmonary emboli. Studies have shown that anticoagulation increases survival rates.

*Copyright © Mometrix Media. You have been licensed one copy of this document for personal use only. Any other reproduction or redistribution is strictly prohibited. All rights reserved.*

- *Diuretics*, such as furosemide (Lasix®) may be needed to relieve edema and restrict fluids, especially with right ventricular hypertrophy.

In some patients who cannot be managed adequately through medical treatment, a heart-lung transplant may be considered as the only effective treatment for long-term survival.

## Pneumonia

Pneumonia is inflammation of the lung parenchyma, filling the alveoli with exudate. It is common throughout childhood and adulthood. Pneumonia may be a primary disease or may occur secondary to another infection or disease, such as lung cancer. It may be caused by bacteria, viruses, parasites, or fungi. Common causes for community-acquired pneumonia (CAP) include:
- *Streptococcus pneumoniae*.
- *Legionella* species.
- *Haemophilus influenzae*.
- *Staphylococcus aureus*.
- *Mycoplasma pneumoniae*.
- Viruses.

Pneumonia may also be caused by chemical damage. Pneumonia is characterized by location:
- **Lobar** involves 1 or more lobes of the lungs. If lobes in both lungs are affected, it is referred to as "bilateral" or "double" pneumonia.
- **Bronchial/lobular** involves the terminal bronchioles, and exudate can involve the adjacent lobules. Usually the pneumonia occurs in scattered patches throughout the lungs.
- **Interstitial** involves primarily the interstitium and alveoli where white blood cells and plasma fill the alveoli, generating inflammation and creating fibrotic tissue as the alveoli are destroyed.

Community-acquired pneumonia:
Community-acquired Methicillin-resistant *Staphylococcus aureus (MRSA)* has emerged as a cause of pneumonia since 1997. Most commonly CA-MRSA presents as skin and soft tissue infections in otherwise healthy young adults or children, most of whom had little contact with healthcare providers in the year prior to the infection. In some patients with soft-tissue infection or exposure from others, cavitous pneumonia can occur very rapidly when superimposed upon a viral infection, such as influenza. The Center for Disease Control (CDC) reported that of 10 cases of influenza-associated CA-MRSA pneumonia in January 2007, 6 died (4 within 4 days). Treatment includes:
- *Trimethoprim-sulfamethoxazole*—1-2 double strength (DS) tablets (160 mg TMP/800 mg SMZ)
- *Minocycline or doxycycline*—100 mg twice daily.
- *Rifampin* in combination (never by itself) with the above antibiotics has a synergistic effect: 300 mg twice daily for 5 days.
- *Vancomycin* intravenously in doses adjusted for individual may be used in severe infections, especially if treatment will exceed 3 weeks, or if there is osteomyelitis.

Hospital-acquired pneumonia:
Rates of hospital-acquired methicillin-resistant *Staphylococcus aureus* (HA-MRSA) have skyrocketed with infection rates in intensive care increasing from 2.1% in 1975 to 55.3% in 2003. Most *Staphylococcus* isolates are now penicillin-resistant, carrying an enzyme that inactivates β-lactam antibiotics, and some are now resistant to vancomycin as well (VRSA). MRSA is endemic in many healthcare facilities, posing a severe risk of systemic, urinary, and pulmonary infections. MRSA is one of the leading causes of hospital-acquired pneumonia, with mortality of 20%. The most important risk factor is intubation and ventilation. Ventilation-associated pneumonia (VAP) occurring within days 1-4 is usually antibiotic sensitive, but those occurring ≥day 5 are usually antibiotic resistant. Cultures obtained with bronchoscopy are more accurate than those from sputum. *Treatment* of choice has been vancomycin, but linezolid has been shown to be more effective, although there

*Copyright © Mometrix Media. You have been licensed one copy of this document for personal use only. Any other reproduction or redistribution is strictly prohibited. All rights reserved.*

is concern that resistance may develop if it is used as a first-line drug.

## Acute bronchitis

Acute bronchitis is an inflammation of the bronchial tree in which swelling and exudate cause a partial obstruction that prevents the lung from fully inflating. Causes include viruses (most common), bacteria, yeasts and fungi, and non-infectious things, such as smoke or air pollutants. In adults, the most common viral triggers are influenza virus, adenovirus, and respiratory syncytial virus (RSV). *Symptoms* vary depending upon cause but may include:

- Dyspnea and tachypnea.
- Cyanosis.
- Heavy productive moist or raspy cough.
- Sputum clear, white, yellow, green, or bloody.
- Localized crackling rales and expiratory high-pitched sibilant wheezes.
- Fever may or may not be present, but a prolonged or high fever may indicate a bacterial infection.

Since most cases of acute bronchitis are caused by viruses and are self-limiting in 2-3 weeks, antibiotics are not helpful, but *treatment* may include:

- Bronchial dilators (albuterol) to improve air exchange.
- Cough suppressant and/or expectorants to relieve cough.
- Antihistamines for those with allergic triggers.
- Antibiotics for bacterial infections.

## Severe acute respiratory syndrome

Severe Acute Respiratory Syndrome (SARS) is caused by a corona virus (Co-V) and presents as a respiratory illness. It is extremely virulent, spreading easily from person to person through close contact by way of contaminated droplets produced by coughing or sneezing. The incubation period is 2-7 days with onset of symptoms at about day 10. SARS has a high mortality rate. Some possibility exists that SARS may also have airborne transmission in some cases with aerosol-producing procedures. High rates of infection have occurred in healthcare workers and others in contact with infected patients. *Symptoms* include:

- Temp >38.0°C, chills, headaches, general malaise.
- Cough, dry and non-productive, dyspnea.
- Myalgia.
- Blood tests show ↓ WBC and platelet counts.

Precautions:

- Negative pressure isolation.
- Full barrier and airborne precautions (recommended by the CDC), especially with aerosol-producing procedures (ventilators, nebulizers, intubation).

*Treatment* is supportive, including oxygen, ventilation, and antipyretics.

## Acute epiglottitis

Acute epiglottitis (supraglottitis) requires immediate medical attention because it can rapidly become obstructive. The onset is usually very sudden; often, it occurs suddenly during the night with a fever but not usually a cough. Because this condition carries a risk of death, immediate treatment is necessary:

| **Symptoms** | *Tripod position*: Person sits upright, leaning forward with chin out, mouth open, and tongue protruding. *Agitation*: Person appears restless, tense, and agitated. *Drooling*: Excess secretions combined with pain or dysphagia and mouth open position cause drooling. *Voice*: Voice sounds thick and "froglike." *Cyanosis*: Color is usually pale and sallow initially progressing to frank cyanosis. *Throat*: Epiglottis bright red and swollen. |
|---|---|

*Copyright © Mometrix Media. You have been licensed one copy of this document for personal use only. Any other reproduction or redistribution is strictly prohibited. All rights reserved.*

| Diagnosis | Direct examination with nasopharyngoscopy. |
|---|---|
| Treatment | Antibiotics for suspected bacterial infections or as indicated by epiglottal cultures. *Respiratory support*, which may require intubation or tracheostomy and mechanical ventilation (especially for viral infection). *Corticosteroids* are usually administered during intubation. |

## Status asthmaticus

Status asthmaticus is a severe acute attack of asthma that does not respond to conventional treatment. An acute attack of asthma is precipitated by some stimulus, such as an antigen that triggers an allergic response, resulting in an inflammatory cascade that causes edema of the mucous membranes (swollen airway), contraction of smooth muscles (bronchospasm), increased mucus production (cough and obstruction), and hyperinflation of airways (decreased ventilation and shunting). Mast cells and T lymphocytes produce cytokines that continue the inflammatory response through increased blood flow coupled with vasoconstriction and bronchoconstriction, resulting in fluid leakage from the vasculature. Epithelial cells and cilia are destroyed, exposing nerves and causing hypersensitivity. Sympathetic nervous system receptors in the bronchi stimulate bronchodilation.

Symptoms:
Status asthmaticus is a severe acute attack of asthma that does not respond to conventional therapy, such as inhaled bronchodilators, and progresses to respiratory failure. The 3 primary *symptoms* of asthma are cough, wheezing, and dyspnea. In cough-variant asthma, a severe cough may be the only symptom, at least initially. The patient with status asthmaticus will often present in acute distress, being non-responsive to inhaled bronchodilators:
- Airway obstruction, sternal and intercostal retractions.

- Tachypnea and dyspnea, increasing cyanosis.
- Forced prolonged expirations.
- Cardiac decompensation with ↑ left ventricular afterload and increased pulmonary edema resulting from alveolar-capillary permeability. Hypoxia may trigger an ↑ in pulmonary vascular resistance with ↑ right ventricular afterload.
- Pulsus paradoxus (decreased pulse on inspiration and increased on expiration), with extra beats on inspiration detected through auscultation but not detected radially. Blood pressure normally decreases slightly during inspiration, but this response is exaggerated.
- Hypoxemia (with impending respiratory failure).
- Hypocapnia followed by hypercapnia (with impending respiratory failure).
- Metabolic acidosis.

Mechanical ventilation:
Mechanical ventilation should be avoided, if possible, because of the danger of increased bronchospasm as well as barotrauma and decreased circulation. Aggressive medical management with β-adrenergic agonists, corticosteroids, and anticholinergics should be tried prior to ventilation. However, there are some absolute indications for the use of intubation and ventilation:
- Cardiac and/or pulmonary arrest.
- Markedly depressed mental status (obtundation).
- Severe hypoxia and/or apnea.
- Bradycardia.

There are a number of other indications that are evaluated on an individual basis and may be an indication for ventilation:
- Exhaustion/muscle fatigue from exertion of trying to breathe.
- Sharply diminished breath sounds and no audible wheezing.
- Pulse paradoxus >20-40 mm Hg. If pulse paradoxus is absent, this is an indication of imminent respiratory arrest.
- $PaO_2$ <70 mm Hg on 100% oxygen.

Copyright © Mometrix Media. You have been licensed one copy of this document for personal use only. Any other reproduction or redistribution is strictly prohibited. All rights reserved.

- Deteriorating mental status.
- Dysphonia.
- Central cyanosis.
- ↑ Hypercapnia, metabolic/respiratory acidosis; pH <7.20.

## Pharmacological agents for asthma

Numerous pharmacological agents are used for control of asthma, some that are long acting to prevent attacks and others that are short-acting to provide relief for acute episodes:

- *β-Adrenergic agonists* include both long-acting and short-acting preparations used for bronchodilation, relaxing smooth muscles, reducing edema, and aiding clearance of mucus. Medications include salmeterol (Serevent), sustained release albuterol (Volmax ER®) and short-acting albuterol (Proventil®) and levalbuterol (Xopenex®).
- *Anticholinergics* aid in preventing bronchial constriction and potentiate the bronchodilating action of β-Adrenergic agonists. The most-commonly used medication is ipratropium bromide (Atrovent®).
- *Corticosteroids* provide anti-inflammatory action by inhibiting immune responses and decreasing edema, mucus, and hyper-responsiveness. Because of numerous side effects, glucocorticosteroids are usually administered orally or parentally for 5 days (prednisone, prednisolone, methylprednisolone) and then switched to inhaled steroids. If a child receives glucocorticoids for more than 5 days, then dosages are tapered. Inhaled corticosteroids include beclomethasone (Vanceril®), budesonide (Pulmicort®) and fluticasone propionate (Flovent®).
- *Methylxanthines* are generally contraindicated for children unless the child is critically ill, in which case they appear to have a role in improving pulmonary function and decreasing the need for mechanical ventilation. Medications include aminophylline and theophylline.

- *Magnesium sulfate* is used to relax smooth muscles and decrease inflammation. If administered intravenously, it must be given slowly to prevent hypotension and bradycardia. Inhaled, it potentiates the action of albuterol.
- *Heliox (helium-oxygen)* is administered to decrease airway resistance to airway obstructions, thereby decreasing respiratory effort. Heliox improves oxygenation for patients being given mechanical ventilation.
- *Leukotriene inhibitors* are used to inhibit inflammation and bronchospasm in long-term management. Medications include montelukast (Singulair®).

## Sleep disordered breathing

Older adults often take longer to fall asleep, awaken more frequently, and sleep less at night and more in the daytime than younger adults. About half of older adults have insomnia and up to 65%-70% have combined sleeping disorders. Sleep disorders include sleep apnea, insomnia, circadian rhythm disorders, and sleep-related movement disorders. Patients may not report sleep disorders but may present with vague complaints of feeling tired, lethargic, and depressed. Sleep disorders may be related to pain, incontinence or urinary frequency, obesity, neurodegenerative diseases, dyspnea, depression, anxiety disorders, bereavement, poor sleep habits, numerous medications (benzodiazepines, antihistamines, antidepressants, diuretics, anti-Parkinson drugs, theophylline, and anticonvulsants), caffeine, and alcohol. Polysomnography (PSG [overnight sleep study]) and sleep diaries may aid diagnosis. *Treatment* includes bright light therapy in the evening to keep people awake, dark room at night, set times for sleeping and arising (avoiding excessive napping), elimination of caffeine, reduced noise at night, increased daytime exercise/activity, treatment of restless leg syndrome (RLS) or sleep apnea, and medical sleep aids, such as sedatives/hypnotics.

*Copyright © Mometrix Media. You have been licensed one copy of this document for personal use only. Any other reproduction or redistribution is strictly prohibited. All rights reserved.*

Obstructive sleep apnea:

Obstructive sleep apnea results from passive collapse of the pharynx during sleep, often associated with narrow or restricted upper airway (micrognathia, obesity, enlarged tonsils). It is more common in middle-aged overweight males and is exacerbated by drinking and ingesting alcohol or sedative drugs before sleeping. *Symptoms* include daytime somnolence, headache, cognitive impairment, depression, personality changes, recent increase in weight, and impotence. Patients often snore loudly with cycles of breath cessation caused by apneic periods up to 60 seconds, occurring at least 30 times a night. ECG changes may indicate bradydysrhythmia during apnea and tachydysrhythmia when breathing resumes. *Diagnosis* is by polysomnography and evaluation of $O_2$ saturation during sleep. Laboratory findings include erythrocytosis. Thyroid function tests should be done to rule out hypothyroidism. *Treatment* includes weight loss, nasal continuous positive airway pressure (CPAP) at night, and surgical repair (uvulopalatopharyngoplasty and/or nasal septoplasty). Supplemental oxygen improves $O_2$ saturation but increases length of apneic periods, and pharmacologic treatment is rarely helpful.

## Lung volume reduction

Lung volume reduction surgery (LVRS) usually involves removing about 20%-35% of lung tissue that is not functioning adequately in order to reduce the lung size so that the lungs work more effectively. This procedure is most commonly used with adult emphysematous COPD patients. In adults, surgery is usually bilateral; however, some patients are not candidates for bilateral surgery because of cardiac disease or emphysema affecting only 1 lung. Unilateral surgery has been shown to be effective. Surgical removal of part of the lung improves ventilation and gas exchange and does not require the immunosuppressive therapy required for lung transplantation. Studies have shown that patients with low risk for the surgery and with emphysematous changes in the upper lobes can benefit from the surgery, but high-risk patients with more wide spread emphysematous changes have increased mortality rates. The surgery may be done through an open-chest thoracotomy or through a less invasive video-assisted thoracotomy.

## Pneumonectomy

Pneumonectomy is surgical removal of 1 of the lungs. There are 2 surgical procedures:
- **Simple**: removal of just the lung.
- **Extrapleural**: removal not only of the lung but also part of the diaphragm on the affected side and the pericardium on that same side.

During the operative procedure, much care must be taken to prevent contamination of the remaining lung, including the use of bronchus blockers or a prone position during surgery. Removal of the lung is indicated for a number of conditions:
- Severe bronchiectasis from chronic suppurative pneumonia, resulting in dilation of terminal bronchioles.
- Severe hypoplasia.
- Unilateral lung destruction with pulmonary hypertension.
- Pulmonary hemorrhage.
- Lobar emphysema.
- Cancerous lesions (the most common reason for surgery).
- Chronic pulmonary infections with destruction of lung tissue.

Because the lung capacity is reduced, persistent shortness of breath may occur with exertion even many months after surgery.

## Lobectomy

Lobectomy removes 1 or more lobes of a lung (which has 2 on the left and 3 on the right) and is usually done for lesions or trauma that is confined to 1 lobe, such as tubercular lesions, abscesses or cysts, cancer (usually non-small cell in early stages), traumatic injury, or bronchiectasis. Surgery is usually done through

*Copyright © Mometrix Media. You have been licensed one copy of this document for personal use only.*
*Any other reproduction or redistribution is strictly prohibited. All rights reserved.*

an open thoracotomy or video-assisted thoracotomy. Complications can include hemorrhage, post-operative infection with or without abscess formation, and pneumothorax. Usually 1-2 chest tubes are left in place in the immediate post-surgical period to remove air and/or fluid.

Segmental resection removes a bronchovascular segment and is used for small lesions in the periphery, i.e., bronchiectasis or congenital cysts or blebs.

Wedge resection removes a small wedge-shaped portion of the lung tissue and is used for small peripheral lesions, granulomas, or blebs.

Bronchoplastic (sleeve) reconstruction removes part of bronchus and lung tissue with reanastomosis of bronchus and is used for small lesions of the carina or bronchus.

## Tracheostomy

Tracheostomy, a surgical tracheal opening, may be utilized for mechanical ventilation. Tracheostomy tubes are inserted into the opening to provide a conduit and maintain the opening. Tracheostomy tubes are usually silastic or plastic, most lacking an inner cannula because they are non-adherent. The tube is secured with ties around the neck. Because the air entering the lungs through the tracheostomy bypasses the warming and moistening effects of the upper airway, air is humidified through a room humidifier or through delivery of humidified air through a special mask or mechanical ventilation. The patient with a tracheostomy must have continuous monitoring of vital signs and respiratory status to ensure patency of tracheostomy. Regular suctioning is needed, especially initially, to remove secretions:

- Suction catheter should be 50% the size of the tracheostomy tube to allow ventilation during suctioning.
- Vacuum pressure: 80-100 mm Hg.
- Catheter should only be inserted ≤ 0.5 cm beyond tube to avoid damage to tissues or perforation.

- Catheter should be inserted without suction and with intermittent suction on withdrawal.

## Conscious sedation

Conscious sedation is used to decrease sensations of pain and awareness caused by a surgical or invasive procedure, such a biopsy, chest tube insertion, fracture repair, and endoscopy. It is also used during presurgical preparations, such as insertion of central lines, catheters, and use of cooling blankets. Conscious sedation uses a combination of analgesia and sedation so that patients can remain responsive and follow verbal cues but have a brief amnesia preventing recall of the procedures. The patient must be monitored carefully, including pulse oximetry, during this type of sedation. The most commonly used drugs include

- Midazolam (Versed®): This is a short-acting water-soluble sedative, with onset of 1-5 minutes, peaking in 30 minutes, and with a duration usually of about 1 hour (but may last up to 6 hours).
- Fentanyl: This is a short-acting opioid with immediate onset, peaking in 10-15 minutes and with duration of about 20-45 minutes.
- The fentanyl/midazolam combination provides both sedation and pain control. Conscious sedation usually requires 6 hours fasting prior to administration.

## *Endocrine*

### Diabetes mellitus

Diabetes mellitus is the most common metabolic disorder in young people, affecting about 1.5 million children and adolescents. Of these, 70%-85% have Type 1 diabetes and the rest have Type 2 diabetes. Over 6% of adults have diabetes, but only two thirds of these have been diagnosed.

| Type | Symptoms | Treatment |
|------|----------|-----------|
| Type I Immune mediated form with insufficient insulin | Pronounced polyuria and polydipsia. Short onset. May be overweight or had recent | Insulin as needed to control blood sugars. Glucose monitoring |

*Copyright © Mometrix Media. You have been licensed one copy of this document for personal use only. Any other reproduction or redistribution is strictly prohibited. All rights reserved.*

| | | |
|---|---|---|
| production because of destruction of pancreatic beta cells. | weight loss. Ketoacidosis present on diagnosis. | 1-4 times daily. Low carbohydrate diet. Exercise. |
| **Type II** Insulin resistant form with defect in insulin secretion. | Long onset. Obese with no weight loss or significant weight loss. Mild or absent polyuria and polydipsia. Ketoacidosis or glycosuria without ketonuria. Androgen-mediated problems such as hirsutism and acne. Hypertension. | Diet and exercise. Glucose monitoring. Oral medications. |

## Hyperglycemia

Hyperglycemia is elevation of serum glucose level ≥180 mg/dL, although symptoms may not be evident until the level reaches ≥270 mg/dL. The most common cause is diabetes mellitus (associated with decreased levels of insulin), but elevations of glucose may also be related to chronic pancreatitis, acromegaly, Cushing's syndrome, and adverse reactions to drugs, such as furosemide, glucocorticoids, growth hormone, oral contraceptives, and thiazides. *Symptoms* of hyperglycemia are similar to symptoms found in chronic diabetes and include ketoacidosis, polyuria, polydipsia, polyphagia, weight loss, and encephalopathy. Stress-related hyperglycemia is common after stroke or myocardial infarction and increases risk of mortality. Physiological stress related to infection may also increase glucose levels. Hyperglycemia can be treated with insulin and by treatment of the underlying cause or by discontinuation of drug administration.

## Ketoacidosis

Ketoacidosis is a complication of diabetes mellitus. Inadequate production of insulin results in glucose being unavailable for metabolism, so lipolysis (breakdown of fat) produces free fatty acids (FFAs) as an alternate fuel source. Glycerol in both fat cells and the liver is converted to ketone bodies (β-hydroxybutyric acid, acetoacetic acid, and acetone), which are used for cellular metabolism but less efficiently than glucose. Excess ketone bodies are excreted in the urine (ketonuria) or exhalations. The ketone bodies lower serum pH, leading to ketoacidosis. *Symptoms* include:

- Kussmaul respirations: hyperventilation to eliminate buildup of carbon dioxide, associated with "ketone breath."
- Fluid imbalance, including loss of potassium and other electrolytes from cellular death, resulting in dehydration and diuresis with excess thirst.
- Cardiac arrhythmias, related to potassium loss, can lead to cardiac arrest.
- Hyperglycemia: blood glucose may vary from 300-800 mg/dL. Normal values for fasting blood glucose: 60-100 mg/dL.

*Treatment* includes:
- Insulin therapy by continuous infusion initially.
- Rehydration and electrolyte replacement.

## Hypoglycemia

Hypoglycemia (low blood sugar) almost always results from treatment for diabetes mellitus, such as the use of insulin. Most often, hypoglycemia is caused by too much medication (insulin or oral medications) and/or inadequate nutritional intake. Excessive exercise, illness, and infections that burn glucose stores can also result in hypoglycemia. Because the brain requires glucose to function, an inadequate supply of glucose can affect the central nervous system. *Symptoms* include:
- Blood glucose <50-60 mg/dL.

*Copyright © Mometrix Media. You have been licensed one copy of this document for personal use only. Any other reproduction or redistribution is strictly prohibited. All rights reserved.*

- Central nervous system: seizures, altered consciousness, lethargy, and poor feeding with vomiting, myoclonus, respiratory distress, diaphoresis, hypothermia, and cyanosis.
- Adrenergic system: diaphoresis, tremor, tachycardia, palpitation, hunger, and anxiety.

*Treatment* depends on identifying and correcting the underlying cause and includes:
- Glucose/Glucagon administration to elevate blood glucose levels.
- Diazoxide (Hyperstat®) to inhibit release of insulin.
- Somatostatin (Sandostatin®) to suppress insulin production.
- Careful monitoring.

## Insulin

There are a number of different types of insulin with varying action times. Insulin is used to metabolize glucose for those whose pancreases do not produce insulin. People may need to take a combination of insulins (short and long-acting) to maintain glucose control. Duration of action may vary according to the individual's metabolism, intake, and level of activity:
- *Humalog* (Lispro H) is a fast acting, short duration insulin that acts within 5-15 minutes, peaking between 45-90 minutes and lasting 3-4 hours.
- *Regular* (R) is a relatively fast acting, 30-minute insulin that peaks in 2-5 hours and last 5-8 hours.
- *NPH* (N) or *Lente* (L)) insulin is intermediate acting with onset in 1-3 hours, peaking at 6-12 hours and lasting 16-24 hours.
- *Ultralente* (U) is a long acting insulin with onset in 4-6 hours, peaking at 8-20 hours, and lasting 24-28 hours.
- *Combined NPH/Regular* (70/30 or 50/50) has an onset of 30 minutes, peaks at 7-12 hours, and lasts 16-24 hours.

## Oral hypoglycemic agents

Oral hypoglycemic agents, also known as sulfonylureas, are used to treat diabetes mellitus, type II. These drugs are derived from sulphonamide and bind to potassium channel receptors, preventing potassium efflux, allowing influx of calcium and release of insulin from pancreatic islets. They are effective in decreasing serum levels of glucagon and potentiating the production of insulin. There are both first-generation drugs and second-generation drugs; the second-generation drugs have shorter half-lives and increased potency over first-generation drugs. First-generation drugs include:
- *Acetohexamide* with half-life of 6-8 hours and duration of 12-18 hours.
- *Chlorpropamide* with half-life of 36 hours and duration of 60 hours.
- *Tolazamide* with half-life of 7 hours and duration of 12-14 hours.
- *Tolbutamide* with half-life of 4.5-6.5 hours and duration of 6-12 hours.

Second-generation drugs include:
- *Glipizide* with half-life of 4 hours and duration of 24 hours.
- *Glyburide* with half-life of 1.5-3.0 hours and duration of 24 hours.

## Serum glucose

Glucose is manufactured by the liver from ingested carbohydrates and is stored as glycogen for use by the cells. If intake is inadequate, glucose can be produced from muscle and fat tissue, leading to increased wasting. High levels of glucose are indicative of diabetes mellitus, which predisposes people to skin injuries, slow healing, and infection. Fasting blood glucose levels are used to diagnose and monitor:
- Normal values: 70-99 mg/dL.
- Impaired: 100-125 mg/dL.
- Diabetes: $\geq 126$ mg/dL.

*Copyright © Mometrix Media. You have been licensed one copy of this document for personal use only. Any other reproduction or redistribution is strictly prohibited. All rights reserved.*

There are a number of different conditions that can increase glucose levels: stress, renal failure, Cushing syndrome, hyperthyroidism, and pancreas disorders. Medications, such as steroids, estrogens, lithium, phenytoin, diuretics, and tricyclic antidepressants, may increase glucose levels. Other conditions, such as adrenal insufficiency, liver disease, hypothyroidism, and starvation, can decrease glucose levels.

## Hemoglobin A1

Hemoglobin A1C comprises hemoglobin A with a glucose molecule because hemoglobin holds onto excess blood glucose, so it shows the average blood glucose levels over a 2-3 month period. It is used primarily to monitor long-term diabetic therapy:
- Normal value: ≤6%.
- Elevation: >7%.

## ADA Recommendations

The American Diabetes Association Clinical Practice Recommendations for the management of diabetes include:
- **Complete evaluation**: Appropriate laboratory testing and history.
- **Management plan**: Development of plan and educational goals and strategies.
- **Glycemic control**: Self-monitoring of blood glucose (3-4 times daily if on multiple insulin injections or insulin pump) and A1C (<7%) twice yearly for patients meeting treatment goals and quarterly for those not meeting goals or with change in therapy.
- **Medications**: Intensive insulin (≥3 insulin injections daily or continuous subcutaneous infusion) or insulin analogs for type 1 diabetes and oral medications for type 2, if needed (after initial insulin [if hyperglycemic]).
- **Diabetes self-management education (DSME):** Education should be provided according to national standards (covering 9 areas of diabetes management) and should include self-management and psychosocial issues in a skill-based approach.
- **Medical nutrition therapy (MNT):** Diet modifications should be individualized and may include low fat, low carbohydrate. Saturated fats should be restricted to <7% of total calories and carbohydrates monitored through use of carbohydrate counting or exchanges. Sugar alcohols and non-nutritive sweeteners (aspartame, Splenda®) may be used. Alcohol intake should be limited to 1 drink per day for females and 2 drinks per day for males.
- **Physical activity:** Aerobic activity ≥150 min/week (ideally 30 minutes daily) to 50%-70% of maximum heart rate and (unless contraindicated) those with type 2 should do resistance training 3 times weekly.
- **Psychosocial assessment and care:** Screening should be done for such issues as depression, eating disorders, financial resources, psychiatric history, and cognitive impairment.
- **Failure to meet treatment goals:** Assessment of barriers to compliance or changes in treatment may be indicated.
- **Intercurrent illness:** Increased monitoring of blood glucose or blood ketones and intervention may be needed to prevent hyperglycemia or hypoglycemia.
- **Hypoglycemia:** Immediate treatment with 15-20 g glucose for conscious patients, repeated in 15 minutes if self-monitored blood glucose indicates continued hypoglycemia. Snack should be eaten when normal glucose level reached. Those at risk should carry glucagon.
- **Immunizations:** Adults should receive 1 lifetime pneumococcal vaccine. In addition, a one-time revaccination should be given to those >65 who had an original injection >5 years ago or who have nephrotic syndrome, chronic renal disease or are immunocompromised. All those ≥6 months of age should have an annual influenza vaccine.

Copyright © Mometrix Media. You have been licensed one copy of this document for personal use only. Any other reproduction or redistribution is strictly prohibited. All rights reserved.

# Hematology/Immunology

## Red blood cells

Red blood cells (RBCs or erythrocytes) are biconcave disks that contain hemoglobin (95% of mass), which carries oxygen throughout the body. The heme portion of the cell contains iron, which binds to the oxygen. RBCs live about 120 days after which they are destroyed and their hemoglobin is recycled or excreted. Normal red blood cell counts vary by sex:

- Males >18 years: 4.5-5.5 million per $mm^3$.
- Females >18 years: 4.0-5.0 million per $mm^3$.

The most common disorders of RBCs are those that interfere with production, leading to various types of anemia:

- Blood loss.
- Hemolysis.
- Bone marrow failure.

The morphology of RBCs may vary depending upon the type of anemia:

- Size: Normocytes, microcytes, macrocytes.
- Shape: Spherocytes (round), poikilocytes (irregular), drepanocytes (sickled).
- Color (reflecting concentration of hemoglobin): Normochromic, hypochromic.

Laboratory tests:
A number of different tests are used to evaluate the condition and production of red blood cells in addition to the red blood cell count:

- Hemoglobin: Carries oxygen and is decreased in anemia and increased in polycythemia. Normal values:
  - o   Males >18 years: 14.0-17.46 g/dl.
  - o   Females >18 years:  12.0-16.0 g/dl.
- Hematocrit: Indicates the proportion of RBCs in a liter of blood (usually about 3 times the hemoglobin number). Normal values:
  - o   Males >18 years:        45%-52%.
  - o   Females >18 years:    36%-48%.
- Mean corpuscular volume (MCV): Indicates the size of RBCs and can differentiate types of anemia. For adults, <80 is microcytic and >100 is macrocytic. Normal values:
  - o   Males >18 years:            84-96 $\mu m^3$.
  - o   Females >18 years:       76-96 $\mu m^3$.
- Reticulocyte count:  measures marrow production and should rise with anemia. Normal values: 0.5-1.5% of total RBCs.

## Anemia

Anemia results in a decrease in oxygen transportation and decreased perfusion throughout the body, causing the heart to compensate by increasing cardiac output. As the blood becomes less viscous, there is decreased peripheral resistance, so more blood is pumped to the heart, and this increased flow can cause turbulence that results in a heart murmur and, if severe or prolonged, heart failure. Anemia is commonly caused by hemorrhage, hemolysis, hematopoiesis, or dietary iron deficiency in women who are menstruating. Children can tolerate low oxygen levels better than adults; however, growth and sexual development may be delayed with chronic anemia. *Symptoms* include:

- General malaise and weakness, poor feeding/anorexia.
- Pallor, shortness of breath on exertion.
- Headache, dizziness, apathy, depression, decreased attention span, slowed thought processes.
- Shock symptoms (with severe blood loss): tachycardia, hypotension, poor peripheral circulation, and pallor.

*Treatment*:

- Treatment of underlying cause.
- Blood or blood components, as indicated.
- Supportive care:  oxygen, intravenous fluids.
- Splenectomy for hemolytic anemias.

Disseminated intravascular coagulation

Disseminated intravascular coagulation (DIC) (consumption coagulopathy) is a secondary disorder that is triggered by another, such as trauma, congenital heart disease, necrotizing

*Copyright © Mometrix Media. You have been licensed one copy of this document for personal use only. Any other reproduction or redistribution is strictly prohibited. All rights reserved.*

enterocolitis, sepsis, and severe viral infections. DIC triggers both coagulation and hemorrhage through a complex series of events that includes trauma that causes tissue factor (transmembrane glycoprotein) to enter the circulation and bind with coagulation factors, triggering the coagulation cascade. This stimulates thrombin to convert fibrinogen to fibrin, causing aggregation and destruction of platelets and forming clots that can be disseminated throughout the intravascular system. These clots increase in size as platelets adhere to the clots, causing blockage of both the microvascular systems and larger vessels, and this can result in ischemia and necrosis. Clot formation triggers fibrinolysis and plasmin to breakdown fibrin and fibrinogen, causing destruction of clotting factors, resulting in hemorrhage. Both processes, clotting and hemorrhage, continue at the same time, placing the patient at high risk for death, even with treatment.

Symptoms and treatment:

The onset of disseminated intravascular coagulation (DIC) symptoms may be very rapid or a slower chronic progression from a disease, such as in children with large vascular malformations. *Symptoms* include:

- Bleeding from surgical or venous puncture sites.
- Bleeding from umbilicus and trachea in newborns.
- Evidence of GI bleeding with distention, bloody diarrhea.
- Hypotension and acute symptoms of shock.
- Petechiae and purpura with extensive bleeding into the tissues.
- Laboratory abnormalities:
  o Prolonged prothrombin and partial prothrombin times.
  o Decreased platelet counts and fragmented RBCs.
  o Decreased fibrinogen.

Those who develop the chronic manifestation of the disease usually have fewer acute symptoms and may slowly develop ecchymosis or bleeding wounds.

*Treatment* varies and includes:

- Identifying and treating underlying cause.
- Replacement blood products, such as platelets and fresh frozen plasma.
- Anticoagulation therapy (heparin) to increase clotting time.
- Cryoprecipitate to increase fibrinogen levels.
- Coagulation inhibitors and coagulation factors.

Laboratory testing:

Disseminated intravascular coagulation (DIC) panel includes a number of tests. Generally, test results that measure materials needed for clotting are decreased and those that measure clotting times are increased. Typical findings that indicate DIC include:

- *Activate partial thromboplastin time (APTT):* Increased time.
- Prothrombin time: Findings vary, may be increased time (in 75% of patients), normal time (25%) or shortened (25%).
- *Partial thromboplastin time:* Increased time (in 50%-60%).
- *Thrombin time:* Increased.
- *D-Dimer:* Increased (usually more reliable than fibrin split products [FSP]): D-dimer is a specific polymer that results when fibrin breaks down, giving a marker to indicate the degree of fibrinolysis.
- *Fibrinogen:* Decreased.
- *Platelets:* <100,000.
- *Fibrin split products (FSP):* Increased (in 75%-100%). FSPs occur as more clots form and more breakdown of fibrinogen and fibrin occurs, interfering with blood coagulation by coating platelets and disrupting thrombin, and also attaching to fibrinogen so stable clots can't form.
- *Clotting factor assays (V, VI, VII, X, XIII):* Decreased.
- *Antithrombin III:* Decreased (in 90%).

## HITTS

Heparin-induced thrombocytopenia and thrombosis syndrome (HITTS) occurs in patients

Copyright © Mometrix Media. You have been licensed one copy of this document for personal use only. Any other reproduction or redistribution is strictly prohibited. All rights reserved.

receiving heparin for anticoagulation. There are 2 types:

- **Type I** is a transient condition occurring within a few days and causing depletion of platelets (<100,000 mm$^3$), but heparin may be continued as the condition usually resolves without intervention.
- **Type II** is an autoimmune reaction to heparin that occurs in 3%-5% of those receiving unfractionated heparin and also occurs with low-molecular weight heparin. It is characterized by low platelets (<50,000 mm$^3$) that are ≥50% below baseline. Onset is 5-14 days but can occur within hours of reheparinization. Death rates are ≤30%. Heparin-antibody complexes form and release platelet factor 4 (PF4), which attracts heparin molecules and adheres to platelets and endothelial lining, stimulating thrombin and platelet clumping. This puts the patient at risk for thrombosis and vessel occlusion rather than hemorrhage, causing stroke, myocardial infarction, and limb ischemia with symptoms associated with the site of thrombosis.

*Treatment* includes:
- Discontinuation of heparin.
- Direct thrombin inhibitors (lepirudin, argatroban).

## ReoPro®-induced coagulopathy

ReoPro® (abciximab) is used to prevent cardiac ischemia for those undergoing percutaneous cardiac intervention. It inhibits the aggregation of platelets. It is used with aspirin and/or weight-adjusted low dose heparin and potentiates the action of anticoagulants. However, its use with non-weight adjusted longer acting heparin can cause thrombocytopenia with increased risk of hemorrhage. This occurs especially with readministration of the drug, which can induce the formation of antibodies and an allergic reaction that is characterized by anaphylaxis and thrombocytopenia. Because of the danger of hemorrhage, ReoPro® is contraindicated if there is active bleeding or a history of bleeding or a

cerebrovascular accident (CVA) within the 2 years prior, history of a CVA, platelet count <100,000 mm$^3$, or a recent history of oral anticoagulation. Careful monitoring of platelet counts prior to administration and the use of weight-adjusted low dose heparin is important to prevent bleeding. Heparin should be discontinued after the percutaneous coronary intervention (PCI).

## Coagulation profile

The coagulation profile measures clotting mechanisms, identifies clotting disorders, screens preoperative patients, and diagnoses excessive bruising and bleeding. Values vary depending on the laboratory:

- **Prothrombin time (PT):** 10 – 14 seconds. Time increases with anticoagulation therapy, vitamin K deficiency, ↓ prothrombin, DIC, liver disease, and malignant neoplasm. Some drugs may shorten time.
- **Partial thromboplastin time (PTT):** 30 – 45 seconds. Increases with hemophilia A & B, von Willebrand's, vitamin deficiency, lupus, DIC, and liver disease.
- **Activate partial thromboplastin time (APTT):** 21 – 35 seconds. Similar to PTT, but decreases in extensive cancer, early DIC, and after acute hemorrhage.
- **Thrombin clotting time (TCT) or Thrombin time (TT):** 7 – 12 seconds (<21). Used most often to determine the dosage of heparin. Prolonged with multiple myeloma, abnormal fibrinogen, uremia, and liver disease.
- **Bleeding time:** 2 – 9.5 minutes. (Using Ivy method on the forearm). Increases with DIC, leukemia, renal failure, aplastic anemia, von Willebrand's, some drugs, and alcohol.
- **Platelet count:** 150 – 400,000. Increased bleeding <50,000 and increased clotting >750,000.

*Copyright © Mometrix Media. You have been licensed one copy of this document for personal use only. Any other reproduction or redistribution is strictly prohibited. All rights reserved.*

# Neurology

## Cranial nerve assessment

The nurse should be familiar with cranial nerve assessment as part of evaluation for suspected head injury/disorder:

I. **Olfactory** (smell): The person is asked to smell and identify a substance, such as coffee or soap, with 1 nostril held closed, and then the exercise if repeated using the other nostril.

II. **Optic** (vision): Test visual acuity and the ability to recognize color. Test each eye separately. Red desaturation is tested by having the person look at a red object with first 1 eye and then the next to determine if the color looks the same with both eyes or is dull with 1 eye.

III. **Oculomotor** (eye muscles and pupil response): Using a penlight, the examiner checks the person's eyes for size, shape, reaction to light and accommodation. Eyes are checked for rotation and conjugate movements. The lids should be examined for ptosis.

IV. **Trochlear** (eye muscles—upward movement): Eye movement is checked by having the person follow a moving finger with the eyes on the vertical plane.

V. **Trigeminal** (chewing muscles, sensory): The person closes his eyes for the sensory examination and is instructed to indicate to the examiner when part of his face is stroked (light stroke with cotton). The forehead, cheek, and jaw are stroked. The same areas are then examined for sensations of sharp or dull. The eye should be observed for blinking and tearing; however touching the cornea with cotton or other items should be avoided because this can cause abrasion. The jaw muscles are assessed by having the person hold the mouth open, as well as palpating the muscles on each side to determine if they are equal in size and strength.

VI. **Abducens** (eye muscles—lateral movement): The person is also asked to follow the finger from the 1-o'clock position clockwise to the 11-o'clock position. At the horizontal and vertical axis, the eyes should be checked for deviation or nystagmus, which may occur normally only in the extreme lateral position.

VII. **Facial nerve** (facial expression, tears, taste, and saliva): Usually, only the motor portion is evaluated for nerve VII, and taste is examined with the testing of cranial nerve IX, but the examiner can test the ability to discriminate between salt and sugar. Motor functions are assessed by asking the person to frown, smile, puff out the cheeks, and wrinkle the forehead. The muscles are observed for symmetry. The person is asked to hold his eyes tightly closed while the examiner attempts to open the lids with her thumb on the lower lid and her index finger on the upper lid, using care not to apply pressure to the eye.

VIII. **Vestibulocochlear** (balance and hearing): Balance is checked with tandem gait and Romberg's test. Hearing is checked (with the person's eyes closed) by rubbing fingers together or holding a ticking watch next to one ear and then the other. Weber's test may be done to evaluate lateralization, along with Rinne's test for bone and air conduction.

  a. **Weber's test:** A vibrating tuning fork is touched to the top of the head or the forehead and the person is asked if the sound is equal in both ears. Hearing deficit in 1 ear suggests sensorineural hearing loss.

  b. **Rinne's test:** A vibrating tuning fork is held on the mastoid bone and the time measured until sound ceases. Then, the vibrating tuning fork is held at the external ear. Sound is normally heard twice as long through air as through bone. If there is conductive hearing loss, the sound is heard longer through the bone. If there is sensorineural hearing loss, the sound is heard longer through the air.

IX. **Glossopharyngeal** (taste, mouth sensation): This test is not usually performed unless the person complains of a lack of taste or abnormalities of taste. The mouth must be moist for accurate assessment, so the person should drink water, if possible, before the test, and the testing substance should be in a

Copyright © Mometrix Media. You have been licensed one copy of this document for personal use only. Any other reproduction or redistribution is strictly prohibited. All rights reserved.

solution. The person is tested for recognition of sweet, sour, bitter, and salt.

X. **Vagus** (swallowing, gag reflex): The examiner has the person open his mouth and say "aw." The uvula and palate should elevate equally on both sides. The gag reflex is usually tested if the person reports difficulty swallowing or changes in speech. Gag reflex is tested by lightly touching the tongue blade to the soft palate. Some people are hyper-responsive, so accurate testing of the gag reflex may be difficult.

XI. **Spinal accessory** (muscle movement—sternocleidomastoid, trapezius): These muscular movements are tested by the examiner placing her hands along the side of the person's face and asking the person to turn the face first to one side and then to the other against resistance. This is done to determine if the person's strength is normal and equal. Then, the examiner places her hands on the person's shoulders and asks the person to shrug the shoulders, elevating them upward, against resistance, to determine if the strength is normal and equal.

XII. **Hypoglossal** (tongue): The examiner asks the person to stick out his tongue to determine if it deviates to one side, indicating a lesion on that side of the brain. To determine if there is equal strength on both sides of the tongue, a tongue blade is held against the side of the tongue, and the person is asked to push against it with the tongue. Both sides are checked to determine if strength is normal and equal.

### Peripheral Nerve assessment

A neurological evaluation should include peripheral nerve assessment to determine if injury has impaired nerve function. Nerves function should be assessed for both sensation and movement. Assessment of sensation is done with a sharp or pointed instrument, using care not to prick the skin. The person should feel a slick prick if the sensory function is intact:

- **Median:** The median nerve branches from the brachial plexus, which arises from C5, C6, C7, C8, and T1. The median nerve travels down the arm and forearm, through the carpal tunnel. Sensation is evaluated by pricking the top or distal surface of the index finger. Movement is evaluated by having the person touch the ends of the thumb and little finger together and having the person flex the wrist.

- **Peroneal:** The peroneal nerve branches from the sciatic nerve, which arises from the L4, L4 and S1, S2, and S3 dorsal nerves and travels down the leg. The peroneal nerve enervates the lower leg, foot, and toes. Sensation is evaluated by pricking the webbed area between the great and second toe. Movement is evaluated by having the person dorsiflex and extend the foot.

- **Radial:** The radial nerve branches from the brachial plexus and enervates the dorsal surface of the arm and hand, including the thumb and fingers 2, 3, and 4. Sensation is evaluated by pricking in skin in the webbed area between the thumb and the index finger. Movement is evaluated by having the person extend the thumb, the wrist, and fingers at the metacarpal joint.

- **Tibial:** The tibial nerve branches from the sciatic nerve. The tibial nerve travels down the back of the leg, through the popliteal fossa at the back of the knee and terminates at the plantar side of the foot. Sensation is evaluated by pricking the medial and lateral aspects of the plantar surface of the foot. Movement is evaluated by having the person plantar flex the toes and then the ankle.

- **Ulnar:** The ulnar nerve branches from the sciatic nerve and travels down the arm from the shoulder, traveling along the anterior forearm beside the ulna, to the palm of the hand. Sensation is evaluated by pricking the distal fat pad at the end of the small finger. Movement is evaluated by having the person extend and spread all fingers.

### Cerebral aneurysms

Cerebral aneurysms, the weakening and dilation of a cerebral artery, are usually congenital (90%), with the remaining (10%) resulting from

Copyright © Mometrix Media. You have been licensed one copy of this document for personal use only. Any other reproduction or redistribution is strictly prohibited. All rights reserved.

direct trauma or infection. Aneurysms usually range from 2-7 mm and occur in the Circle of Willis at the base of the brain. A rupturing aneurysm may decrease perfusion as well as increasing pressure on surrounding brain tissue. Cerebral aneurysm are classified as follows:

- **Berry/saccular:** The most common congenital type occurs at a bifurcation and grows from the base on a stem, usually at the Circle of Willis.
- **Fusiform:** Large and irregular (>2.5 cm) and rarely ruptures but causes increased intracranial pressure. Usually involves the internal carotid or vertebrobasilar artery.
- **Mycotic:** Rare type that occurs secondary to bacterial infection and a septic embolus.
- **Dissecting:** Wall is torn apart and blood enters layers. This may occur during angiography or secondary to trauma or disease.
- **Traumatic Charcot-Bouchard (pseudoaneurysm):** Small lesion resulting from chronic hypertension.

## Arteriovenous malformation

Arteriovenous malformation (AVM) is a congenital abnormality described as a tangle of dilated arteries and veins without a capillary bed. AVMs can occur anywhere in the brain and may cause no significant problems. Usually the AVM is "fed" by 1 or more cerebral arteries, which enlarge over time, shunting more blood through the AVM. The veins also enlarge in response to increased arterial blood flow because of the lack of a capillary bridge between the two. Because vein walls are thinner and lack the muscle layer of an artery, the veins tend to rupture as the AVM becomes larger, causing a subarachnoid hemorrhage. Chronic ischemia that may be related to the AVM can result in cerebral atrophy. Sometimes small leaks, usually accompanied by headache and nausea and vomiting, may occur before rupture. AVMs may cause a wide range of neurological *symptoms*, including changes in mentation, dizziness, sensory abnormalities, confusion, and dementia. *Treatment* includes:

- Supportive management of symptoms.

- Surgical repair or focused irradiation (definitive treatments).

## Subarachnoid hemorrhage

Subarachnoid hemorrhage (SAH) may occur after trauma but is common from rupture of a berry aneurysm or an arteriovenous malformation (AVM). However, there are a number of disorders that may be implicated: neoplasms, sickle cell disease, infection, hemophilia, and leukemia. The first presenting symptom may be complaints of severe headache, nausea and vomiting, nuchal rigidity, palsy related to cranial nerve compression, retinal hemorrhages, and papilledema. Late complications include hyponatremia and hydrocephalus.

*Symptoms* worsen as intracranial pressure rises. SAH from aneurysm is classified as follows:

- Grade I: No symptoms or slight headache and nuchal rigidity.
- Grade II: Moderate-severe headache with nuchal rigidity and cranial nerve palsy.
- Grade III: Drowsy, progressing to confusion or mild focal deficits.
- Grade IV: Stupor, with hemiparesis (moderate-severe), early decerebrate rigidity, and vegetative disturbances.
- Grade V: Coma state with decerebrate rigidity.

*Treatment* includes:

- Identifying and treating underlying cause.
- Observing for re-bleeding.
- Anti-seizure medications (such as Dilantin®) to control seizures.
- Antihypertensives.
- Surgical repair, if indicated.

## Intracranial hemorrhage

Hemorrhage is always a concern with head trauma because even injuries that appear slight can result in vascular rupture, resulting in hemorrhage between the skull and the brain. There are 2 types of hemorrhage that often

*Copyright © Mometrix Media. You have been licensed one copy of this document for personal use only. Any other reproduction or redistribution is strictly prohibited. All rights reserved.*

occur from head trauma: epidural and subdural. **Epidural** hemorrhage is bleeding between the dura and the skull, pushing the brain downward and inward. The hemorrhage is usually caused by arterial tears, so bleeding is often rapid, leading to severe neurological deficits and respiratory arrest. Initially, the body compensates by rapidly absorbing cerebrospinal fluid and decreasing blood flow, but the compensatory measure is soon overwhelmed. The most common site is the parietotemporal region, forcing the medial part of the temporal lobe under the tentorial edge, compressing nerves and vessels. This type of injury usually results from skull fractures with middle meningeal artery lacerations or venous bleeding, such as may occur with a blow to the head from a fall or a motor vehicle accident.

## Subdural hemorrhage

Subdural hemorrhage is bleeding between the dura and the cerebrum, usually from tears in the cortical veins of the subdural space. It tends to develop more slowly than epidural hemorrhage and can result in a subdural hematoma. If the bleeding is acute and develops within minutes or hours of injury, the prognosis is poor. Subacute hematomas that develop more slowly cause varying degrees of injury. Subdural hemorrhage is a common injury related to trauma, but it can result from coagulopathies or aneurysms. Symptoms of acute injury may occur within 24-48 hours, but subacute bleeding may not be evident for up to 2 weeks after injury. Chronic hemorrhage occurs primarily in the elderly. *Symptoms* vary and may include bradycardia, tachycardia, hypertension, and alterations in consciousness. Older children and adults usually require surgical evacuation of the hematoma.

## Seizure disorders

Seizures are sudden involuntary abnormal electrical disturbances in the brain that can manifest as alterations of consciousness, spastic tonic and clonic movements, convulsions, and loss of consciousness. Seizures may be partial, affecting part of the brain or generalized, affecting the whole brain. Seizures are a symptom of underlying pathology. Many seizures are transient. Some seizures may result from pathology, such as meningitis, cerebral edema, brain trauma, or brain tumors. Others are idiopathic, predisposing the person to recurrent seizures, usually of the same type. Seizures are believed caused by cells known as epileptogenic focus, which increase electrical discharge in response to physiological changes, such as fatigue or changes in blood sugar level. The electrical discharge spreads to the brainstem, causing generalized seizures. Seizures are characterized as focal (localized), focal with rapid generalization (spreading), and generalized (widespread). Seizure disorders with onset in childhood <4 years usually cause more neurological damage than those that have a later onset.

Partial seizures:
Partial seizures are caused by an electrical discharged to a localized area of the cerebral cortex, such as the frontal, temporal, or parietal lobes with seizure characteristics related to the area of involvement. They may begin in a focal area and become generalized, often preceded by an aura.

- **Simple partial:** Unilateral motor symptoms including somatosensory, psychic, and autonomic.
  - o Aversive: Eyes and head turned away from focal side.
  - o Sylvan (usually during sleep): Tonic-clonic movements of the face, salivation, and arrested speech.
- **Special sensory:** Various sensations (numbness, tingling, prickling, or pain) spreading from 1 area. May include visual sensations, posturing, or hypertonia. Rare for patients <8 years.
- **Complex (Psychomotor):** No loss of consciousness, but altered consciousness and non-responsive with amnesia. May involve complex sensorium with bad tastes, auditory or visual hallucinations, feeing of déjà vu, and strong fear. May carry out repetitive activities, such as walking, running, smacking lips, chewing, or drawling.

*Copyright © Mometrix Media. You have been licensed one copy of this document for personal use only. Any other reproduction or redistribution is strictly prohibited. All rights reserved.*

Rarely aggressive. Seizure usually followed by prolonged drowsiness and confusion. Occurs age 3 through adolescence.

Generalized seizures:
Generalized seizures lack a focal onset and appear to involve both hemispheres, usually presenting with loss of consciousness and no preceding aura.

- **Tonic-clonic (Grand Mal):** Occurs without warning.
  - o Tonic period (10-30 seconds): Eyes roll upward with loss of consciousness, arms flexed, muscles stiffen in symmetric tonic contraction of body, apneic with cyanosis and salivating.
  - o Clonic period (10 seconds to 30 minutes, but usually 30 seconds). Violent rhythmic jerking with contraction and relaxation. May be incontinent of urine and feces. Contractions slow and then stop.
  - o Following seizures, there may be confusion and disorientation, also impairment of motor activity, speech, and vision for several hours. Headache, nausea, and vomiting may occur. The person often falls asleep and awakens conscious.
- **Absence (Petit Mal):** Onset between ages 4-12 and usually ends in puberty. Onset is abrupt with brief loss of consciousness for 5-10 seconds and slight loss of muscle tone, but the person often appears to be daydreaming. Lip smacking or eye twitching may occur.

## Status epilepticus

Status epilepticus (SE) is usually generalized tonic-clonic seizures that are characterized by a series of seizures with intervening time too short for regaining of consciousness. The constant assault and periods of apnea can lead to exhaustion, respiratory failure with hypoxemia and hypercapnia, cardiac failure, and death. There are a number of causes of SE:

- Uncontrolled epilepsy or non-compliance with anticonvulsants.

- Infections, such as encephalitis.
- Encephalopathy or brain attack.
- Drug toxicity (isoniazid). Brain trauma.
- Neoplasms. Metabolic disorders.

*Treatment* includes:

- Anticonvulsants usually beginning with fast-acting benzodiazepine (Ativan®), often in steps, with administration of medication every 5 minutes until seizures subside.
- If cause is undetermined, acyclovir and ceftriaxone may be administered.
- If there is no response to the first 2 doses of anticonvulsants (refractory SE), rapid sequence intubation (RSI), which involves sedation and paralytic anesthesia, may be done while therapy continues. Combining phenobarbital and benzodiazepine can cause apnea, so intubation may be necessary.
- Phenytoin and phenobarbital are added.

## Ischemic strokes

Strokes (brain attacks, cerebrovascular accidents) result when there is an interruption of the blood flow to an area of the brain. The 2 basic types are ischemic and hemorrhagic. About 80% of strokes are ischemic, resulting from blockage of an artery supplying the brain:

- **Thrombosis** in a large artery, usually resulting from atherosclerosis, may block circulation to a large area of the brain. The most common occurrence is in the elderly. Thrombosis may occur suddenly or after episodes of transient ischemic attacks.
- **Lacunar infarct** (penetrating thrombosis in small artery) is more common in those with diabetes mellitus and/or hypertension.
- **Embolism** travels through the arterial system and lodges in the brain, most commonly in the left middle cerebral artery. An embolism may be cardiogenic, resulting from cardiac arrhythmia or surgery. An embolism usually occurs rapidly with no warning signs.
- **Cryptogenic** has no identifiable cause.

*Copyright © Mometrix Media. You have been licensed one copy of this document for personal use only. Any other reproduction or redistribution is strictly prohibited. All rights reserved.*

Medical management:

Medical management of ischemic strokes with tissue plasminogen activator (tPA, Activase®), the primary treatment, should be initiated within 3 hours of the event:

- **Thrombolytic medication** (tPA) is produced by recombinant DNA and is used to dissolve fibrin clots. It is given intravenously (0.9 mg/kg up to 90 mg) with 10% injected as an initial bolus and the rest over the next hour.
- **Antihypertensives** if MAP >130 mm Hg or systolic BP >220 mm Hg.
- **Cooling** to reduce hyperthermia.
- **Osmotic diuretics** (mannitol), hypertonic saline, loop diuretics (Lasix®), and/or corticosteroids (dexamethasone) to ↓ cerebral edema and intracranial pressure.
- **Aspirin/anticoagulation** may be used with embolism.
- **Stool softeners** to prevent constipation.
- **Monitor and treat hyperglycemia.**

Contraindications to thrombolytic therapy include:

- Evidence of cerebral or subarachnoid hemorrhage or other internal bleeding or history of intracranial hemorrhage.
- Recent stroke, head trauma, or surgery.
- Uncontrolled hypertension, seizures.
- Intracranial AVM, neoplasm, or aneurysm.
- Current anticoagulation therapy.
- Low platelet count (<100,000 mm³).

## Hemorrhagic strokes

Hemorrhagic strokes account for about 20% and result from a ruptured cerebral artery, causing not only lack of oxygen and nutrients but also edema that causes widespread pressure and damage:

- **Intracerebral** is bleeding into the substance of the brain from an artery in the central lobes, basal ganglia, pons, or cerebellum. Intracerebral hemorrhage usually results from atherosclerotic degenerative changes, hypertension, brain tumors, anticoagulation therapy, or some illicit drugs, such as crack

and cocaine. Stroke onset is often sudden and may cause death.

- **Intracranial aneurysm** occurs with ballooning cerebral artery ruptures, most commonly at the Circle of Willis.
- **Arteriovenous malformation** (AVM) is a tangle of dilated arteries and veins without a capillary bed. This is a congenital abnormality. Rupture of AVMs is a cause of brain attack in young adults.
- **Subarachnoid hemorrhage** is bleeding in the space between the meninges and brain, resulting from aneurysm, AVM, or trauma. This type of hemorrhage compresses brain tissue.

## Strokes

Strokes most commonly occur in the right or left hemisphere, but the exact location and the extent of brain damage affects the type of presenting symptoms. If the frontal area of either side is involved, there tends to be memory and learning deficits. Some symptoms are associated with specific areas and help to identify the area involved:

- Right hemisphere: This results in left paralysis or paresis and a left visual field deficit that may cause spatial and perceptual disturbances. For example, people may have difficulty judging distance. Fine motor skills may be impacted, resulting in trouble dressing or handling tools. People may become impulsive and exhibit poor judgment, often denying impairment. Left-sided neglect (lack of perception of things on the left side) may occur. Depression is common as well as short-term memory loss and difficulty following directions. Language skills usually remain intact.
- **Left hemisphere:** This type of stroke results in right paralysis or paresis and a right visual field defect. Depression is common, and people often exhibit slow, cautious behavior, requiring repeated instruction and reinforcement for simple tasks. Short-term memory loss and difficulty learning new material or understanding generalizations is common. Difficulty with mathematics,

Copyright © Mometrix Media. You have been licensed one copy of this document for personal use only. Any other reproduction or redistribution is strictly prohibited. All rights reserved.

reading, writing, and reasoning may occur. Aphasia (expressive, receptive, or global) is common.

- **Brain stem**: Because the brain stem controls respiration and cardiac function, a brain attack frequently causes death, but those who survive may have a number of problems, including respiratory and cardiac abnormalities. Strokes may involve motor or sensory impairment or both.
- **Cerebellum**: This area controls balance and coordination. Strokes in the cerebellum are rare but may result in ataxia, nausea and vomiting, headaches, dizziness, or vertigo.

# Gastrointestinal
## Gastrointestinal hemorrhage

Gastrointestinal (GI) hemorrhage may occur in the upper or lower gastrointestinal track. The primary cause (50%-70%) of GI hemorrhage is peptic ulcer disease (gastric and duodenal ulcers), which results in deterioration of the gastro mucosal lining, compromising the glycoprotein mucous barrier and the gastroduodenal epithelial cells that provide protection from gastric secretions. The secretions literally digest the mucosal and submucosal layers, damaging blood vessels and causing hemorrhage. The primary causes are NSAIDs and infection with *Helicobacter pylori*. *Symptoms* include:

- Abdominal pain and distention.
- Hematemesis.
- Bloody or tarry stools.
- Hypotension with tachycardia.

*Treatment* includes:

- Fluid replacement with transfusions if necessary.
- Antibiotic therapy for *Helicobacter pylori*.
- Endoscopic thermal therapy to cauterize or injection therapy (hypertonic saline, epinephrine, ethanol) to cause vasoconstriction.
- Arteriography with intraarterial infusion of vasopressin and/or embolizing agents, such

as stainless steel coils, platinum microcoils, or Gelfoam pledgets.
- Vagotomy and pyloroplasty if bleeding persists.

## Stress-related erosive syndrome

Stress-related erosive syndrome (SRES [stress ulcers]) occurs most frequently in patients who are critically ill, such as those with severe or multi-organ trauma, mechanical ventilation, sepsis, severe burns, and head injury with increased intracranial pressure. Stress induces changes in the gastric mucosal lining and decreased perfusion of the mucosa, causing ischemia. SRES involves hemorrhage in ≥30% of cases with mortality rates of 30%-80%, so prompt identification and treatment is critical. The lesions tend to be diffuse, so they are more difficult to treat than peptic ulcers. *Symptoms* include:

- Coffee ground emesis.
- Hematemesis.
- Abdominal discomfort.

*Treatment* includes prophylaxis in those at risk:

- Sucralfate (Carafate®) protects mucosa against pepsin.
- Famotidine (Pepcid®), nizatidine (Axid®), ranitidine (Zantac®) or cimetidine (Tagamet®) reduces gastric secretions.

*Treatment* for active bleeding includes:

- Intraarterial infusion of vasopressin.
- Intraarterial embolization.
- Oversewing of ulcers or total gastrectomy if bleeding persists.

## Esophageal varices

Esophageal varices are torturous dilated veins in the submucosa of the esophagus (usually the distal portion), a complication of cirrhosis of the liver in which obstruction of the portal vein causes an increase in collateral vessels, a decrease in circulation to the liver, and an increase in pressure in the collateral vessels in the submucosa of the esophagus and stomach.

*Copyright © Mometrix Media. You have been licensed one copy of this document for personal use only. Any other reproduction or redistribution is strictly prohibited. All rights reserved.*

This causes the vessels to dilate. Because they tend to be fragile and inelastic, they tear easily, causing sudden massive esophageal hemorrhage. Bleeding from varices occurs in 19%-50% of cases with associated mortality rates of 40%-70%. *Treatment* may include:

- Fluid and blood replacement.
- Intravenous vasopressin, somatostatin, and octreotide to ↓ portal venous pressure and provide vasoconstriction.
- Endoscopic injection with sclerosing agents.
- Endoscopic variceal band ligation.
- Esophagogastric balloon tamponade to apply direct pressure.
- Transjugular intrahepatic portosystemic shunting (TIPS) creates a channel between systemic and portal venous systems to reduce portal hypertension. A variety of other shunts may be done surgically if bleeding persists.

**Diverticulosis and diverticulitis**

Diverticulosis is a condition in which diverticula (saclike pouchings of the bowel lining that extend through a defect in the muscle layer) occur anywhere within the GI tract. Diverticulitis occurs as diverticula become inflamed when food or bacteria are retained within diverticula. This may result in abscess, obstruction, perforation, bleeding, or fistula. *Symptoms* are similar to appendicitis and include:

- Steady pain in left lower quadrant (sigmoid diverticulitis).
- Change in bowel habits.
- Tenesmus.
- Dysuria from irritation.
- Toxic reactions: fever, severe pain, leukocytosis.
- Recurrent urinary infections from fistula.
- Paralytic ileus from peritonitis or intraabdominal irritation.

Diagnosis is per CT, as barium enema will show diverticula but not inflammation. *Treatment* includes:

- Rehydration and electrolytes per intravenous fluids.

- Nothing by mouth initially.
- Antibiotics, broad spectrum (IV if toxic reactions).
- Nasogastric (NG) suction if necessary for obstruction.
- Careful observation for signs of perforation or obstruction.

**Peritonitis**

Peritonitis (inflammation of the peritoneum) may be primary (from infection of blood or lymph) or, more commonly, secondary, related to perforation or trauma of the gastrointestinal tract. Common causes include perforated bowel, ruptured appendix, abdominal trauma, abdominal surgery, peritoneal dialysis or chemotherapy, or leakage of sterile fluids, such as blood, into the peritoneum. *Symptoms* of peritonitis are those of an acute abdomen:

- Diffuse abdominal pain with rebound tenderness (Blumberg's sign).
- Abdominal rigidity.
- Paralytic ileus.
- Fever (with infection).
- Nausea and vomiting.
- Sinus tachycardia.

*Diagnosis* is made according to clinical presentation, abdominal x-rays, which may show distention of the intestines or air in the peritoneum, and laboratory findings, such as leukocytosis. Blood cultures may indicate sepsis. *Treatment* includes:

- Intravenous fluids and electrolytes.
- Broad-spectrum antibiotics.
- Surgical consultation for laparoscopy, as indicated, to determine cause of peritonitis and effect repair.

**Cholecystitis**

Cholecystitis can result in obstruction of the bile duct related to calculi as well as to pancreatitis from obstruction of the pancreatic duct. The disease is more common in overweight women 20-40 years but can occur in pregnant women and people of all ages, especially those who are

- 68 -

*Copyright © Mometrix Media. You have been licensed one copy of this document for personal use only. Any other reproduction or redistribution is strictly prohibited. All rights reserved.*

diabetic or elderly. Children may develop cholecystitis secondary to cystic fibrosis, obesity, or total parenteral nutrition. *Symptoms* range from asymptomatic to severe right upper quadrant or epigastric pain, persisting 2-6 hours per episode. Disease of the biliary tract may cause radiation of pain to the back and nausea and vomiting. Cholangitis may result in jaundice and altered mental status. *Diagnosis* is confirmed by ultrasound, as laboratory findings may be within the normal range. *Treatment* includes:

- Antibiotics for sepsis or ascending cholangitis.
- Antispasmodic agents (glycopyrrolate) for biliary colic and vomiting.
- Analgesics (meperidine for acute pain).
- Antiemetics (promethazine).
- Surgical consultation to determine if laparoscopic or open cholecystectomy is warranted.

## Irritable bowel syndrome

Irritable bowel syndrome is a chronic disorder characterized by abdominal discomfort and change in bowel habits. It is more common in females (66%) than males and may be associated with depression and history of bacterial gastroenteritis. Symptoms are often vague but usually do not include sudden onset, fever, nocturnal diarrhea, or weight loss. Typical symptoms include:

- Abdominal pain relieved by defecation.
- Change in frequency of defecation, which may occur more frequently (>3 times daily) or less frequently (<3 times weekly).
- Change in character of stool from very hard to very loose and watery.
- Difficulty with defecation involving straining, urgency, or inability to completely evacuate rectum.
- Abdominal distention.

*Diagnosis* is based on symptoms and laboratory tests to rule out other disorders (such as celiac disease). *Treatment* includes reducing stressors, dietary management (reducing fatty foods, caffeine, and foods that cause flatulence), medications (antispasmodics, antidiarrheals, laxatives, tricyclic antidepressants, serotonin receptor agonists and antagonists, nonabsorbable antibiotics (rifaximin 400 mg three times daily), and cognitive therapy for relaxation.

## Gastroesophageal reflux disease

Gastroesophageal reflux disease (GERD) is involuntary regurgitation of stomach contents into the esophagus, usually caused by decreased tone in the gastroesophageal valve and hiatal hernia, causing damage to the mucosal lining of the esophagus. Chronic esophagitis, strictures, Barrett's esophagus (abnormal changes in cells of distal esophagus), and esophageal cancer may develop. GERD *symptoms* include:

- Epigastric pain and "heartburn," dysphagia.
- Chronic cough, especially at night, and hoarseness.
- Earache.
- Sinusitis.

*Treatment* includes:

- Avoiding large meals or after dinner snacking and eating at least 3 hours before going to bed or lying down.
- Modifying food intake to avoid coffee, alcohol, fatty food, spicy foods, and cruciferous vegetables.
- Sleeping with head of the bed elevated and on left side.
- Medications include histamine-2 receptor blockers (famotidine and ranitidine), proton pump inhibitors, alginic acid (Gaviscon®), and antacids (without aluminum).
- Surgical repair (fundoplication) may be needed if medical treatment is not adequate.

## Dysphagia

Dysphagia occurs in about 10% of noninstitutionalized older adults and even more in hospitalized patients. Difficulty swallowing is evident with solids (meat, bread) and thin liquids. There are a variety of causes:

- Stroke: About 30% have dysphagia.

*Copyright © Mometrix Media. You have been licensed one copy of this document for personal use only. Any other reproduction or redistribution is strictly prohibited. All rights reserved.*

- Neuromuscular diseases: Parkinson's disease, myasthenia gravis, multiple sclerosis, and ALS.
- Drugs: Phenothiazines.
- Dementia: Patients may not chew food adequately or may forget to swallow.
- Achalasia (failure of the esophagus to contract effectively and sphincter to relax).
- Esophageal stricture, diverticulum, or web (from iron deficiency) and cancer.
- Esophageal cancer.

*Symptoms* include chest tightness or pain, regurgitation, choking, esophageal reflux (especially when supine), and aspiration pneumonia. Weight loss and dehydration may result. *Diagnosis* is based on symptoms, barium swallow, and endoscopy. *Treatment* includes diagnosing and treating underlying causes, sitting upright to eat, avoiding eating before lying down, chewing foods carefully and sipping water after swallowing, thickening thin liquids, using smaller table utensils to limit bite-size, strengthening exercises, and taking medications to relax the esophagus.

## Bowel obstruction

Bowel obstruction occurs when there is a mechanical obstruction of the passage of intestinal contents because of constriction of the lumen, occlusion of the lumen, or lack of muscular contractions (paralytic ileus). Obstruction may be caused by congenital or acquired abnormalities/disorders. *Symptoms* include:
- Abdominal pain and distention.
- Abdominal rigidity.
- Vomiting and dehydration.
- Diminished or no bowel sounds.
- Severe constipation (obstipation).
- Respiratory distress from diaphragm pushing against pleural cavity.
- Shock as plasma volume diminishes and electrolytes enter intestines from bloodstream.
- Sepsis as bacteria proliferates in bowel and invade bloodstream.

## Bowel infarction

Bowel infarction is ischemia of the intestines related to severely restricted blood supply. It can be the result of a number of different conditions, such as strangulated bowel or occlusion of arteries of the mesentery, and may follow untreated bowel obstruction. People present with acute abdomen and shock, and mortality rates are very high even with resection of an infarcted bowel.

## Paralytic ileus

Paralytic ileus is the lack of intestinal contractions and bowel sounds because of paralysis of the bowel caused by excessive manipulation during surgery (most common), prolonged period of anesthesia, infection (such as peritonitis and appendicitis), or narcotic pain medications. *Symptoms* resemble those of bowel obstruction although the intestines remain patent:
- Constipation and lack of flatulence.
- Abdominal distention.
- Nausea and vomiting.
- Diffuse abdominal discomfort.
- Lack of bowel sounds on auscultation.

Patients should be encouraged to exercise and roll from side to side frequently to stimulate contractions. Ileus may require IV fluids and nasogastric tube to decompress the stomach and prevent vomiting until normal bowel activity returns. Oral foods/fluids should be avoided. Most cases resolve within a few days, but contrast studies should be done if the ileus is prolonged to rule out mechanical obstruction.

## Short gut syndrome

Short gut (bowel) syndrome occurs when removal of part of the small intestine results in a malabsorptive condition. *Symptoms* relate to the amount of bowel removed and the area of resection:
- Resection of the terminal ileum interferes with absorption of bile salts and vitamin B12. If <100 cm removed, malabsorption of

*Copyright © Mometrix Media. You have been licensed one copy of this document for personal use only. Any other reproduction or redistribution is strictly prohibited. All rights reserved.*

bile salts causes watery diarrhea. Treatment includes salt binding resins (cholestyramine 2 to 4 g three times daily). If >100 cm removed, steatorrhea with resultant malabsorption of fat-soluble vitamins occurs. Additional treatment includes low fat diet, vitamins, and calcium supplements to prevent oxalate kidney stone.

- Resection of >40%-50% of small bowel results in weight loss, diarrhea, and electrolyte imbalance. If colon and 100 cm of proximal jejunum are retained, a low fat, high complex carbohydrate diet, and electrolytes may maintain nutrition, but if the colon is removed, 200 cm of jejunum is required for adequate nutrition. Otherwise, parenteral nutrition is required, and this can lead to liver failure and death or liver/intestine transplantation.

## Ulcerative colitis

Ulcerative colitis is superficial inflammation of the mucosa of colon and rectum, causing ulcerations in the areas where inflammation has destroyed cells. These ulcerations, ranging from pinpoint to extensive, may bleed and produce purulent material. The mucosa of the bowel becomes swollen, erythematous, and granular. Onset of ulcerations is usually between ages 15 and 30, and there is a genetic component. Ulcerative colitis may affect only the rectum (ulcerative proctitis), the entire colon (pancolitis), or only the left colon (limited or distal colitis).

*Symptoms*:
- *Abdominal pain* may be absent or mild unless severe disease.
- *Bloody diarrhea/rectal bleeding* in absence of infection may result in anemia and fluid and electrolyte depletion. Diarrhea becomes more frequent as colonic involvement increases.
- *Fecal urgency and tenesmus* may occur.
- *Anorexia* resulting in weight loss and fatigue.
- *Systemic disorders* with eye inflammation, arthritis, liver disease, and osteoporosis as

the immune system triggers generalized inflammation.

*Treatment:*
- Aminosalicylates.
- Steroids.
- Immunomodulatory agents.
- Antispasmodics.
- Iron supplementation.
- High protein diet with decreased fiber.

## Crohn's disease

Crohn's disease manifests with inflammation of the GI system. Inflammation is transmural (often leading to intestinal stenosis and fistulas), focal and discontinuous with aphthous ulcerations progressing to linear and irregular shaped ulcerations. Granulomas may be present. Common sites of inflammation are the terminal ileum and cecum. Condition is usually chronic, but an acute flare-up may mimic appendicitis. Children may have delayed development and stunted growth. There is a genetic component to the disease.

*Symptoms*:
- *Perirectal abscess/fistula* in advanced disease.
- *Diarrhea* usually present with colonic disease. May have nocturnal bowel movements, watery stools, and rectal hemorrhage.
- *Anemia* may develop with chronic bleeding.
- *Abdominal pain,* commonly occurring in lower right quadrant, usually indicates transmural inflammation; may include post-prandial pain and cramping.
- *Other symptoms* include nausea and vomiting (usually related to strictures of small intestine), weight loss (with small intestine involvement), fever, and night sweats.

*Treatment* includes:
- Corticosteroids and antibiotics for acute exacerbations.
- Immunomodulatory agents (cyclosporine, methotrexate).
- Antidiarrheals.

*Copyright © Mometrix Media. You have been licensed one copy of this document for personal use only. Any other reproduction or redistribution is strictly prohibited. All rights reserved.*

## Cirrhosis

Cirrhosis is a chronic hepatic disease in which normal liver tissue is replaced by fibrotic tissue that impairs liver function. There are 3 types:

- **Alcoholic** (from chronic alcoholism) is the most common type and results in fibrosis about the portal areas. The liver cells become necrotic, replaced by fibrotic tissue, with areas of normal tissue projecting in between, giving the liver a hobnail appearance.
- **Postnecrotic** has broad bands of fibrotic tissue, resulting from acute viral hepatitis.
- **Biliary**, the least common type, is caused by chronic biliary obstruction and cholangitis, with resulting fibrotic tissue about the bile ducts.

Cirrhosis may be either compensated or decompensated. **Compensated** cirrhosis usually involves non-specific symptoms, such as intermittent fever, epistaxis, ankle edema, indigestion, abdominal pain, and palmar erythema. Hepatomegaly and splenomegaly may also be present.

Decompensated cirrhosis:
Decompensated cirrhosis occurs when the liver can no longer adequately synthesize proteins, clotting factors, and other substances so that portal hypertension occurs. *Symptoms* include:

- Hepatomegaly, portal obstruction resulting in jaundice and ascites.
- Chronic elevated temperature.
- Purpura resulting from thrombocytopenia, with bruising and epistaxis.
- Bacterial peritonitis may develop with ascites.
- Esophageal varices.
- Edema of extremities and presacral area resulting from reduced albumin in the plasma.
- Vitamin deficiency from interference with formation, use, and storage of vitamins, such as A, C, and K.
- Anemia from chronic gastritis and ↓ dietary intake.

- Hepatic encephalopathy with alterations in mentation.
- Hypotension.
- Atrophy of gonads.

*Treatment* varies according to the symptoms and is supportive rather than curative because the fibrotic changes in the liver cannot be reversed: Dietary supplements and vitamins; diuretics (potassium sparing), such as Aldactone® and Dyrenium®, to decrease ascites; colchicine to reduce fibrotic changes; and liver transplant, which is the definitive treatment.

## Hepatic failure

Hepatic failure occurs when the liver is no longer able to function. The liver receives oxygenated blood from the right and left hepatic arteries and blood rich in nutrients from the intestinal tract through the portal vein. Portal venous blood is normally filtered in the liver, and pathogens and nutrients are absorbed and metabolized by hepatocytes. Nutrients are stored in the liver or excreted into the hepatic veins and inferior vena cava. With liver failure, this process is impaired by **portal hypertension**: The portal vein that feeds the liver becomes obstructed, reducing blood flow and increasing blood pressure in the portal venous system, already compressed by cirrhotic changes. The liver cannot filter blood adequately, and the increased pressure creates collateral blood vessels that bypass the obstruction, returning unfiltered blood to the systemic circulation as a result. Collateral vessels cause varices to form in the esophagus or other areas. Increased aldosterone causes sodium and fluid retention. Plasma albumin decreases, causing fluid to leak from the vascular system and resulting in ascites.

These conditions are part of the syndrome of liver failure:
- **Hepato-renal syndrome** results in marked decrease in renal blood flow with resultant increase in azotemia (nitrogenous substances). Sodium levels fall and potassium increases, and there are multiple abnormalities in blood chemistries and

*Copyright © Mometrix Media. You have been licensed one copy of this document for personal use only. Any other reproduction or redistribution is strictly prohibited. All rights reserved.*

clotting times. Hepato-renal syndrome is often related to hepatic encephalopathy.

- **Hepatic encephalopathy** occurs when ammonia crosses the blood-brain barrier and is absorbed by brain tissue. Normally, when protein is digested in the intestines, the ammonia that is produced as a byproduct is filtered by the liver and metabolized to form urea. When blood flow from the portal system is restricted, the serum ammonia level increases. Ammonia causes increasing confusion, stupor, and coma with marked changes in EEG.

## Fulminant hepatitis

Fulminant hepatitis/liver failure is a severe life-threatening acute liver infection. It may be triggered by hepatitis or other viruses, toxins (carbon tetrachloride), Wilson's disease, and drugs--most commonly, Tylenol® (acetaminophen), a drug frequently used by teenagers for suicide attempts. Fulminant hepatitis has a very rapid onset with jaundice, hepatic necrosis, hepatic encephalopathy, coma, and death often within days. However, in some cases, liver failure may be delayed. It is classified according to the time to liver failure:

- Hyperacute: 0-7 days.
- Acute: 8-28 days.
- Subacute: 28-72 days.

Symptoms vary but anorexia is common. Intracranial pressure increases as encephalopathy and cerebral edema occur, and this can result in brainstem compression. As the condition worsens, coagulopathies may cause gastrointestinal bleeding. Renal failure occurs with electrolyte imbalances. Sepsis often leads to multi-organ failure, and death occurs in 80% of patients.

## Liver function studies

Liver function studies include:

| | |
|---|---|
| **Bilirubin** | Determines the ability of the liver to conjugate and excrete bilirubin: direct 0.0-0.3 mg/dL, total 0.0-0.9 mg/dL, and urine 0. |
| **Total protein** | Determines if the liver is producing protein in normal amounts: 7.0-7.5 g/dL: *Albumin*: 4.0-5.5 g/dL. *Globulin*: 1.7=3.3 g/dL. *Serum protein electrophoresis* is done to determine the ratio of proteins. *Albumin/globulin (A/G) ratio*: 1.5:1 to 2.5:1. (Albumin should be greater than globulin). |
| **Pro-thrombin time** | 100% or 12-16 seconds. PT ↑ with liver disease. |
| **Alkaline phosphatase** | 17-142 µ/L in adults. (Normal values vary with method.) Indicates biliary tract obstruction if no bone disease |
| **AST (SGOT)** | 10-40 units. (↑ in liver cell damage.) |
| **ALT (SGPT)** | 5-35 units. (↑ in liver cell damage.) |
| **GGT, GGTP** | 5-55 µ/L females, 5-85 µ/L males. (Increases with alcohol abuse.) |
| **LDH** | 100-200 units. (Increases with alcohol abuse.) |
| **Serum ammonia** | 150-250 mg/dL (Increases in liver failure.) |

## Indicators of malnutrition

There are a number of indicators of malnutrition:

- **Hypermetabolism** resulting from various diseases, such as AIDS, trauma, stress, or infection.
- **Weight loss,** especially sudden or a loss of 10% of normal weight over a 3-month period.

*Copyright © Mometrix Media. You have been licensed one copy of this document for personal use only. Any other reproduction or redistribution is strictly prohibited. All rights reserved.*

- **Low body weight** of <90% of ideal body weight for age.
- **Low Body Mass Index** (BMI) <18.5.
- **Immunosuppressive drugs** that interfere with absorption of nutrients.
- **Malabsorption** of nutrients caused by diseases, such as chronic failure of kidneys or liver.
- **Changes in appetite** that decrease intake of nutrients.
- **Food intolerances**, such as lactose intolerance, resulting from the lack of enzymes needed to completely digest food so that it can be absorbed into the blood stream from the small intestine.
- **Dietary restrictions**, such as limiting of protein with kidney failure.
- **Functional limitations**, such as inability to feed oneself.
- **Lack of teeth or dentures**, limiting intake.
- **Alterations of taste or smell** that render food unpalatable.

Physical assessment:
The physical assessment is an important part of nutritional assessment to determine malnutrition or problems with self-feeding:
- **Hair** may be dry and brittle or thinning.
- **Skin** may show poor turgor, ecchymosis, tears, pressure areas, ulcerations, abrasions, or other compromises.
- **Mouth** may show dry mucous membranes. Lips may have cheilosis, cracking at the corners, and scaly lips (riboflavin deficiency). Gums may be swollen or bleeding, teeth loose or needing care, or dentures poorly fitting. Tongue may be inflamed, dry, cracked, or have sores.
- **Nails** may become brittle. Spoon shaped or pale nail bed indicates low iron.
- **Hands** may be crippled or arthritic, making eating difficult.
- **Vision** may be compromised so that people can't see to prepare food or have difficulty feeding themselves.
- **Mental status** may be impaired to the point that people can't understand diet instructions or prepare or eat meals.

- **Motor skills** may decrease, including hand-mouth coordination or ability to hold utensils.

Types of malnutrition:
Protein malnutrition (kwashiorkor or hypoalbuminemia), inadequate protein but adequate fats and carbohydrates, can result from chronic diarrhea, renal disease, infection, hemorrhage, burns, traumatic injuries, or other illnesses. Onset is usually rapid with loss of visceral protein while skeletal muscle mass is retained, so it may be difficult to detect on a physical exam. *Symptoms* include:
- Hypoalbuminemia and anemia.
- Edema.
- Delayed healing of wound.
- Immuno-incompetence.

Protein-calorie malnutrition (marasmus), inadequate protein and calories, is usually more obvious. Visceral protein is usually intact, as is immune function, because weight loss is gradual. However, patients are often very thin or emaciated from loss of skeletal muscle mass. Many are elderly and have chronic illnesses. *Symptoms* include:
- Decreased basal metabolism.
- Lack of subcutaneous fat, tissue turgor.
- Bradycardia.
- Hypothermia.

Mixed protein-calorie malnutrition (combination) is common in hospitalized patients and has an acute onset with low visceral protein as well as rapid loss of weight, skeletal muscle mass, and fat.

**Starvation**

In response to wounds/illness, the stress response causes a hypermetabolic state, and caloric and protein needs increase markedly at the same time that intake decreases, leading to periods of starvation:
- A short period can result in increased nitrogen in urine and increased output with rapid loss of muscle and weight.

Copyright © Mometrix Media. You have been licensed one copy of this document for personal use only. Any other reproduction or redistribution is strictly prohibited. All rights reserved.

- A prolonged period results in slower weight and muscle loss but can lead to metabolic acidosis with increased ammonia in urine and decreased nitrogen.
- An extended period becomes premorbid with obvious cachexia and weight loss. The midarm muscle circumference decreases, and there are increases in creatinine/height index and urinary urea, as well as decreases in serum albumin, transferrin, and lymphocytes.

## Excessive intake

Excessive intake may cause obesity, which delays wound healing, but it does not necessarily mean nutrition is adequate. Overweight people can still have inadequate protein, vitamins, and minerals. Because protein and caloric requirements for healing are tied to weight, nutritional needs are high, but fat stores help people to tolerate prolonged periods of starvation.

## Nutritional assessment tools

The MNA® (Mini-Nutritional Assessment) by Nestle Nutrition is designed for nutritional assessment of those over age 65 and is only valid for that population. It is a screening and assessment tool to determine the risk for malnutrition and comprises 15 questions about dietary habits and 4 measurements, including Body Mass Index (BMI) using height and weight and mid-arm and calf circumference.

The Nutritional Screening Initiative® is another tool designed for geriatric patients. The interviewer records dietary information as well as social and environmental factors, such as whether the person eats alone, prepares meals, drinks alcohol, and has sufficient income.

The Subjective Global Assessment® assesses nutritional status by a thorough history and physical examination. The history assesses weight change, dietary intake, gastro-intestinal symptoms, and functional impairment. The results of this assessment tool are evaluated subjectively by an experienced interviewer and scores assigned to determine malnutrition risks on a scale of normal to severe.

## Body Mass Index

The Body Mass Index (BMI) formula is a measurement that uses height and weight as an indicator of obesity/malnutrition. This cannot be used alone to diagnose obesity because body types differ. Women often have more body fat than men. Tables are available to make calculations simple, but the BMI can be calculated manually:
- BMI formula using pounds and inches:
  - $BMI = \dfrac{\text{weight in pounds} \times 703}{\text{height in inches}^2}$
- BMI formula using kilograms and meters:
  - $BMI = \dfrac{\text{weight in kilograms}}{\text{height in meters}^2}$

Resulting scores for adults age 20 and over are interpreted according to this chart:
- Below 18.5 Underweight.
- 18.5-24.9   Normal weight.
- 25.0-29.9   Overweight.
- 30 and above        Obese.

The BMI for those under age 20 uses age-sex specific charts pro-vided by the CDC, containing a curved line that indicates percentiles. Criteria for obesity based on these charts and BMI for age <20 follow:
- <5th percentile - Underweight.
- 85th-<95 percentile - At risk for overweight.
- ≥95th percentile - Overweight.

## Nutritional intake routes

Oral intake of nutrition is optimal, and every effort should be made to ensure that those who are able to take oral foods are assisted to do so. This may require complete or partial assistance with feeding. Finger foods may encourage some patients (such as older adults) to eat, and dietary supplements may improve nutrition.

*Copyright © Mometrix Media. You have been licensed one copy of this document for personal use only. Any other reproduction or redistribution is strictly prohibited. All rights reserved.*

Enteral (NG) feeding tubes may be used for short-term (such as after a stroke), but long-term use, especially for those in nursing homes or at end of life, is controversial. While feeding tubes can provide adequate fluids and nutrition, feeding tubes can cause irritation, and aspiration may occur. Gastrostomy tubes may be inserted for long-term feedings.

Total parenteral nutrition (TPN) may be used for those with severe nutritional deficiencies related to inadequate diet, radiotherapy, or chemotherapy, or after surgery, but TPN poses the risk of infection and glucose intolerance and is not advised for long-term administration, especially in older adults.

**Nutritional lab monitoring**

Total protein:
Total protein levels can be influenced by many factors, including stress and infection, but it may be monitored as part of an overall nutritional assessment. Protein is critical for general health and wound healing, and because metabolic rate increases in response to a wound, protein needs increase:
- Normal values:  5-9 g/dL.
- Diet requirements for wound healing:  1.25-1.5 g/kg per day.

Albumin:
Albumin is a protein that is produced by the liver and is a necessary component for cells and tissues. Levels decrease with renal disease, malnutrition, and severe burns. Albumin levels are the most common screening to determine protein levels. Albumin has a half-life of 18-20 days, so it is sensitive to long-term protein deficiencies more than short-term.
- Normal values:     3.5-5.5 g/dL.
- Mild deficiency: 3-3.5 g/dL.
- Moderate deficiency: 2.5-3.0 g/dL.
- Severe deficiency: <2.5 g/dL.

Levels below 3.2 correlate with increased morbidity and death. Dehydration (poor intake, diarrhea, or vomiting) elevates levels, so adequate hydration is important to ensure meaningful results.

Prealbumin:
Prealbumin (transthyretin) is most commonly monitored for acute changes in nutritional status because it has a half-life of only 2-3 days. Prealbumin is a protein produced in the liver, so it is often decreased with liver disease. Oral contraceptives and estrogen can also decrease levels. Levels may rise with Hodgkin's disease or the use of steroids or NSAIDS. Prealbumin is necessary for transportation of both thyroxine and vitamin A throughout the body, so if levels fall, both thyroxine and vitamin A utilization are also affected:
- Normal values: 16-40 mg/dL.
- Mild deficiency: 10-15 mg/dL.
- Moderate deficiency: 5-9 mg/dL.
- Severe deficiency: <5 mg/dL.

Prealbumin is a good measurement because it quickly decreases when nutrition is inadequate and rises quickly in response to increased protein intake. Protein intake must be adequate to maintain levels of prealbumin. Death rates increase with any decrease in prealbumin levels.

Transferrin:
Transferrin, which transports about one third of the body's iron, is a protein produced by the liver. It transports iron from the intestines to the bone marrow where it is used to produce hemoglobin. The half-life of transferrin is about 8-10 days. It is sometimes used as a measure of nutritional status; however, transferrin levels are sensitive to many different things. Levels rapidly decrease with protein malnutrition. Liver disease and anemia can also depress levels, but a decrease in iron, commonly found with inadequate protein, stimulates the liver to produce more transferrin, which increases its levels but also decreases production of albumin and prealbumin. Levels may also increase with pregnancy, use of oral contraceptives, and polycythemia. Thus, transferrin levels alone are not always reliable measurements of nutritional status:
- Normal values:     200-400 mg/dL.

*Copyright © Mometrix Media. You have been licensed one copy of this document for personal use only. Any other reproduction or redistribution is strictly prohibited. All rights reserved.*

- Mild deficiency: 150-200 mg/dL.
- Moderate deficiency: 100-150 mg/dL.
- Severe deficiency: <100 mg/dL.

Total lymphocyte count:
The immune system responds quickly to changes in protein intake because proteins are critical to antibody and lymphocyte production. T-lymphocytes develop in the thymus gland and are a part of the cell-mediated immune response. B-lymphocytes develop in the bone marrow and are part of the humoral (antibody-mediated) immune response. Total lymphocyte count (TLC) can reflect changes in nutritional status because a decrease in protein causes decreased immunity. Lymphocytes are expressed on a differential as a percentage of the white blood count. The TLC is calculated by multiplying the percentage by the total white blood count and then dividing by 100:

- Normal values:      2000 cells/mm$^3$.
- Mild deficiency: 1500-1800 cells/mm$^3$.
- Moderate deficiency: 900-1500 cells/mm$^3$.
- Severe deficiency: <900 cells/mm$^3$.

While low levels may be indicative of malnutrition, levels are also depressed with stress, autoimmune diseases, chemotherapy, infection, and HIV.

Hydration:
Hydration is essential for proper health, healing, and for meaningful results of laboratory measures of nutrition. A number of different tests can be used to monitor hydration:

- **Serum sodium** measures the sodium level in the blood. Some drugs, such as steroids, laxatives, contraceptives, NSAIDS, and IV fluids containing sodium can elevate levels. Other drugs, such as diuretics and vasopressin, can reduce levels.
  - Normal values: 135-150 mEq/L.
  - Dehydration: >150 mEq/L.
- **Serum osmolality** measures the concentration of ions, such as sodium, chloride, potassium, glucose, and urea in the blood. Levels increase with dehydration, which stimulates the antidiuretic hormone (AD), resulting in increased water reabsorption and more concentrated urine in an effort to compensate. Changes in osmolality can affect normal cell functioning, eventually destroying the cells if levels remain high.
  - Normal levels: 285-295 mill-osmoles per kilogram/$H_2O$.
  - Dehydration: >295 mill-osmoles per kilogram/$H_2O$.

**Acute pancreatitis**

Acute pancreatitis is related to chronic alcoholism or cholelithiasis in 90% of patients. Pancreatitis may be triggered by a variety of drugs. Pain is usually acute and may be in mid-epigastric, left upper abdominal, or more generalized. Nausea and vomiting as well as abdominal distention may be present. Complications may include shock, acute respiratory distress syndrome, and multi-organ failure. *Diagnostic* tests include:

- Serum lipase >2 X normal value.
- Serum amylase (less accurate than lipase).
- CT with contrast to determine if there is pancreatic necrosis.
- Ultrasound to check bile duct for obstruction.
- MR cholangiopancreatography may be used in place of CT and ultrasound, where available.

*Treatment* is usually supportive, with oral intake restricted to clear liquids. Rehydration with intravenous fluids may be needed. Biliary obstruction needs to be removed with cholecystectomy. Antibiotics are given if necrosis is related to infection. Analgesia may be indicated.

## *Renal*
**Acute renal failure**

Acute renal failure is an abrupt and almost complete failure of kidney function with decreased glomerular filtration rate (GFR), occurring over a period of hours/days. It most commonly occurs in hospitalized patients but

Copyright © Mometrix Media. You have been licensed one copy of this document for personal use only. Any other reproduction or redistribution is strictly prohibited. All rights reserved.

may occur in others as well. The BUN increases and nitrogenous wastes are retained (azotemia). There are 3 primary categories, related to cause:

- **Prerenal disorders,** such as myocardial infarction, heart failure, sepsis, anaphylaxis, and hemorrhage result in hypoperfusion of the kidney and ↓ GFR.
- **Intrarenal disorders** include burns, trauma, infection, transfusion reactions, and nephrotoxic agents that cause damage to glomeruli or kidney tubules, such as acute tubular necrosis. Burns and crush trauma injuries release myoglobin and hemoglobin from tissues, causing renal toxicity and/or ischemia. With transfusion reactions, hemolysis occurs, and the broken-down hemoglobin concentrates and precipitates in tubules. Medications, such as NSAIDs and ACE inhibitors, may interfere with kidney function by causing hypoperfusion and ischemia.
- **Post renal** involves distal obstruction that increases pressure in tubules and ↓ GFR.

## Acute tubular necrosis

Acute tubular necrosis (ATN) occurs when a hypoxic condition causes renal ischemia that damages tubular cells of the glomeruli, so they are unable to adequately filter the urine, leading to acute renal failure. Causes include hypotension, hyperbilirubinemia, sepsis, surgery (especially cardiac or vascular), and birth complications. ATN may result from nephrotoxic injury related to obstruction or drugs, such as chemotherapy drugs (acyclovir) and antibiotics (sulfonamides and streptomycin). *Symptoms* may be non-specific initially and include life-threatening complications:

- Lethargy.
- Nausea and vomiting.
- Hypovolemia with low cardiac output and generalized vasodilation.
- Fluid and electrolyte imbalance leading to hypertension, CNS abnormalities, metabolic acidosis, arrhythmias, edema, and congestive heart failure.

- Uremia leading to destruction of platelets and bleeding, neurological deficits, and disseminated intravascular coagulopathy (DIC).

*Treatment* includes:

- Identifying and treating the underlying cause.
- Supportive care. Loop diuretics (in some cases), such as Lasix®.
- Antibiotics for infection. Discontinuation of nephrotoxic agents. Kidney dialysis.

## Electrolyte imbalances

Sodium:
Sodium (Na) regulates fluid volume, osmolality, acid-base balance, and activity in the muscles, nerves and myocardium. It is the primary cation (positive ion) in extracellular fluid (ECF), necessary to maintain the ECF levels that are needed for tissue perfusion:

- Normal value: 135-145 mEq/L.
- Hyponatremia: <135 mEq/L.
- Hypernatremia: >145 mEq/L.

| *Hyponatremia* | May result from inadequate sodium intake or excess loss, through diarrhea, vomiting, or NG suctioning. It can occur as the result of illness, such as severe burns, fever, SIADH, and ketoacidosis. **Symptoms** vary: Irritability to lethargy and alterations in consciousness. Cerebral edema with seizures and coma. Dyspnea to respiratory failure. *Treatment:* Identify and treat the underlying cause and provide Na replacement. |
|---|---|
| *Hypernatremia* | May result from renal disease, diabetes insipidus, and fluid depletion. *Symptoms* include irritability to lethargy to confusion to coma, seizures, flushing, muscle weakness and spasms, and thirst. *Treatment* |

Copyright © Mometrix Media. You have been licensed one copy of this document for personal use only. Any other reproduction or redistribution is strictly prohibited. All rights reserved.

| | includes identifying and treating the underlying cause, monitoring Na levels carefully, and IV fluid replacement. |
|---|---|

Potassium:

Potassium (K) is the primary electrolyte in intracellular fluid (ICF) with about 98% inside cells and only 2% in ECF, although this small amount is important for neuromuscular activity. K influences activity of the skeletal and cardiac muscles. K level is dependent upon adequate renal functioning because 80% is excreted through the kidneys and 20% through the bowels and sweat:

- Normal values:   3.5-5.5 mEq/L.
- Hypokalemia:   <3.5 mEq/L.

| **Hypokalemia** | Caused by loss of K through diarrhea, vomiting, gastric suction, and diuresis, alkalosis, decreased K intake with starvation, and nephritis. *Symptoms* include |
|---|---|
| | - Lethargy and weakness.
- Nausea and vomiting.
- Paresthesias.
- Dysrhythmias with ECG abnormalities:  PVCs, flattened T waves.
- Muscle cramps with hyporeflexia.
- Hypotension.
- Tetany.

*Treatment:*  Identify and treat the underlying cause and replace K. |

Potassium excess:

| **Hyperkalemia** >5.5 mEq/L. | Caused by renal disease, adrenal insufficiency, metabolic acidosis, severe dehydration, burns, hemolysis, and trauma. It rarely occurs without renal disease but may be induced by treatment (such as NSAIDs and potassium-sparing diuretics). Untreated renal failure results in reduced excretion. Those with Addison's disease and deficient adrenal hormones suffer sodium loss that results in potassium retention. The primary *symptoms* relate to the effect on the cardiac muscle:

Ventricular arrhythmias with increasing changes in EKC leading to cardiac and respiratory arrest.

Weakness with ascending paralysis and hyperreflexia. Diarrhea. Increasing confusion.

*Treatment* includes identifying underlying cause and discontinuing sources of increased K:

Calcium gluconate to decrease cardiac effects.

Sodium bicarbonate shifts K into the cells temporarily.

Insulin and hypertonic dextrose shift K into the cells temporarily.

Cation exchange resin (Kayexalate®) to decrease K.

Peritoneal dialysis or hemodialysis |
|---|---|

Calcium:

More than 99% of calcium (Ca) is in the skeletal system with 1% in serum, but it is important for transmitting nerve impulses and regulating muscle contraction and relaxation, including the

*Copyright © Mometrix Media. You have been licensed one copy of this document for personal use only. Any other reproduction or redistribution is strictly prohibited. All rights reserved.*

myocardium. Calcium activates enzymes that stimulate chemical reactions and has a role in coagulation of blood:

- Normal values: 1.15-1.34 mg/dL.
- Hypocalcemia: <1.15 mg/dL.
- Hypercalcemia: >1.34 mg/dL.

| | |
|---|---|
| *Hypocalcemia* | May be caused by hypoparathyroidism and occurs after thyroid and parathyroid surgery, pancreatitis, renal failure, inadequate vitamin D, alkalosis, magnesium deficiency and low serum albumin. ***Symptoms*** include Tetany, tingling, seizures, altered mental status. Ventricular tachycardia. *Treatment*: Calcium replacement and vitamin D. |
| *Hypercalcemia* | May be caused by acidosis, kidney disease, hyperparathyroidism, prolonged immobilization, and malignancies. Crisis carries a 50% mortality rate. ***Symptoms*** include: Increasing muscle weakness with hypotonicity. Anorexia, nausea and vomiting. Constipation. Bradycardia and cardiac arrest. ***Treatment***: Identify and treat the underlying cause, loop diuretics, and IV fluids. |

Phosphorus:
Phosphorus, or phosphate, ($PO_4$) is necessary for neuromuscular and red blood cell function, the maintenance of acid-base balance, and providing structure for teeth and bones. About 85% is in the bones, 14% in soft tissue, and <1% in ECF.

- Normal values: 2.4 – 4.5 mEq/L
- Hypophosphatemia: <2.4 mEq/L.
- Hyperphosphatemia: >4.5 mEq/L.

| | |
|---|---|
| *Hypo-phospha-temia* | Occurs with severe protein-calorie mal-nutrition; excess antacids with magnesium, calcium or albumin; hyperventilation; severe burns; and diabetic ketoacidosis. ***Symptoms*** include: Irritability, tremors, seizures and coma. Hemolytic anemia. Decreased myocardial function. Respiratory failure. ***Treatment***: Identify and treat the underlying cause and replace phosphorus. |
| *Hyper-phospha-temia* | Occurs with renal failure, hypoparathyroidism, excessive intake, neoplastic disease, diabetic ketoacidosis, muscle necrosis, and chemotherapy. ***Symptoms*** include: Tachycardia. Muscle cramping, hyperreflexia, and tetany. Nausea and diarrhea. ***Treatment***: Identify and treat the underlying cause, correct hypocalcemia, and provide antacids and dialysis. |

Magnesium:
Magnesium (Mg) is the second most common intracellular electrolyte (after potassium) and activates many intracellular enzyme systems. Mg is important for carbohydrate and protein metabolism, neuromuscular function, and cardiovascular function, producing vasodilation and directly affecting the peripheral arterial system: Normal values: 1.4 mEq/L.
Hypomagnesemia: <1.4 mEq/L.
Hypermagnesemia: >1.4 mEq/L.

| | |
|---|---|
| *Hypomag-nesemia* | Occurs with chronic diarrhea, chronic renal disease, chronic pancreatitis, excess diuretic or laxative use, hyperthyroidism, hypoparathyroidism, severe |

*Copyright © Mometrix Media. You have been licensed one copy of this document for personal use only. Any other reproduction or redistribution is strictly prohibited. All rights reserved.*

| | burns, and diaphoresis. **Symptoms** include: Neuromuscular excitability/tetany. Confusion, headaches and dizziness, seizure and coma. Tachycardia with ventricular arrhythmias. Respiratory depression. **Treatment**: Identify and treat the underlying cause, provide magnesium replacement. |
|---|---|
| **Hyper-magnesemia** | Occurs with renal failure or inadequate renal function, diabetic ketoacidosis, hypothyroidism, and Addison's disease. **Symptoms** include muscle weakness, seizures, dysphagia with de-creased gag reflex, and tachycardia with hypotension. **Treatment**: Identify and treat the cause, IV hydration with calcium, and dialysis. |

Fluid balance:
Body fluid is primarily intracellular fluid (ICF) or extracellular fluid (ECF). By 3 years of age, the fluid balance has stabilized and remains so throughout adulthood:
- ECF: 20%-30% (intrastitial fluid, plasma, transcellular fluid).
- ICF: 40%-50% (fluid within the cells)

The fluid compartments are separated by semipermeable membranes that allow fluid and solutes (electrolytes and other substances) to move by osmosis. Fluid also moves through diffusion, filtration, and active transport. In fluid volume deficit, fluid is out of balance and ECF is depleted; an overload occurs with increased concentration of sodium and retention of fluid. Signs of fluid deficit include:
- Thirsty, restless to lethargic.
- Increasing pulse rate, tachycardia.
- Fontanels depressed (infants).
- ↓ Urinary output.

- Normal BP progressing to hypotension.
- Dry mucous membranes.
- 3%-10% ↓ in body weight.

**Metabolic and respiratory acidosis**

**Pathophysiology:** Metabolic: Increase in fixed acid and inability to excrete acid or loss of base, with compensatory increase of $CO_2$ excretion by lungs. Respiratory: Hypoventilation and $CO_2$ retention, with renal compensatory retention of bicarbonate ($HCO_3$) and increased excretion of hydrogen.

**Laboratory:** Metabolic: Increase in fixed acid and inability to excrete acid or loss of base, with compensatory increase of $CO_2$ excretion by lungs. Respiratory: ↓ Serum pH and ↓ $PCO_2$, $HCO_3$ normal if compensated and ↓ if uncompensated.
Urine pH <6 if compensated.

**Causes:** Metabolic: Diabetic ketoacidosis (DKA), lactic acidosis, diarrhea, starvation, renal failure, shock, and renal tubular acidosis. Respiratory: COPD, overdose of sedative or barbiturate, obesity, severe pneumonia/atelectasis, muscle weakness (Guillain-Barré), and mechanical hypoventilation.

**Symptoms:** Metabolic: Neuromuscular: drowsiness, confusion, headache, coma. Cardiac: ↓ BP, arrhythmias, flushed skin.
GI: nausea, vomiting, abdominal pain, diarrhea. Respiratory: deep inspired tachypnea.
Respiratory: Neuromuscular: drowsiness, dizziness, headache, coma, disorientation, seizures. Cardiac: ↓ BP, VF, flushed skin. GI: absent. Respiratory: hypoventilation with hypoxia.

**Metabolic and respiratory alkalosis**

**Pathophysiology:** Metabolic: Decreased strong acid or increased base, with compensatory $CO_2$ retention by lungs. Respiratory: Hyperventilation and increased excretion of $CO_2$, with compensatory $HCO_3$ excretion by kidneys.

*Copyright © Mometrix Media. You have been licensed one copy of this document for personal use only. Any other reproduction or redistribution is strictly prohibited. All rights reserved.*

**Laboratory:** Metabolic: ↑ Serum pH. $PCO_2$ normal if uncompensated and ↑ if compensated. ↑ $HCO_3$ Urine pH >6 if compensated. Respiratory: ↑ Serum pH. ↓ $PCO_2$ $HCO_3$ normal if uncompensated and ↓ if compensated. Urine pH >6 if compensated.

**Causes:** Metabolic: Excessive vomiting, gastric suctioning, diuretics, potassium deficit, excessive mineralocorticoids, and $NaHCO_3$ intake. Respiratory: Hyperventilation associated with hypoxia, pulmonary embolus, exercise, anxiety, pain, and fever. Encephalopathy, septicemia, brain injury, salicylate overdose, and mechanical hyperventilation.

**Symptoms:** Metabolic: Neuromuscular: dizziness, confusion, nervousness, anxiety, tremors, muscle cramping, tetany, tingling, and seizures. Cardiac: tachycardia and arrhythmias. GI: nausea and vomiting, anorexia. Respiratory: compensatory hypoventilation. Respiratory: Neuromuscular: light-headed, confused, and lethargic. Cardiac: tachycardia and arrhythmias. GI: epigastric pain, nausea and vomiting. Respiratory: hyperventilation.

### Renal function studies

Renal function studies include:

| | |
|---|---|
| **Specific gravity** | 1.015-1.025. Determines kidney's ability to concentrate urinary solutes. |
| **Osmolality (urine)** | 300-900 mOsm/kg/24 hours. Shows early defects if kidney's ability to concentrate urine is impaired. |
| **Osmolality (serum)** | 275-295 mOsm/kg. |
| **Uric acid** | Varies according to age and sex. Levels increase with renal failure. |
| **Creatinine clear-ance (24-hour)** | Varies widely according to age and sex, and decreases with age. Evaluates the amount of blood cleared of creatinine in 1 minute. Approximates the glomerular filtration rate. |

| | |
|---|---|
| **Serum creatinine** | 0.6-1.2 mg/dL. Increases with impaired renal function, urinary tract obstruction, and nephritis. Level should remain stable with normal functioning. |
| **Blood urea nitrogen (BUN)** | 7-8 mg/dL (8-20 mg/dL >age 60). Increase indicates impaired renal function, as urea is end product of protein metabolism. |
| **BUN/ Creatinine ratio** | 10:1. Increases with hypovolemia. With intrinsic kidney disease, the ratio is normal, but the BUN and creatinine are increased. |

### End-stage renal disease

End-stage renal disease (ESRD) occurs when the kidneys are unable to filter and excrete wastes, concentrate urine, and maintain electrolyte balance because of hypoxic conditions, kidney disease, or obstruction in the urinary tract. It results first in azotemia (increase in nitrogenous waste in the blood) and then in uremia (nitrogenous wastes cause toxic symptoms). When >50% of the functional renal capacity is destroyed, the kidneys can no longer carry out necessary functions, and progressive deterioration begins over months or years. Symptoms are often non-specific in the beginning with loss of appetite and energy. *Symptoms* and complications include:

- Weight loss.
- Headaches, muscle cramping, general malaise.
- ↑ Bruising and dry or itching skin.
- ↑ BUN and creatinine, sodium and fluid retention with edema.
- Hyperkalemia, calcium and phosphorus depletion, resulting in altered bone metabolism, pain, and retarded growth.
- Metabolic acidosis.
- Anemia with decreased production of RBCs.
- Increased risk of infection.
- Uremic syndrome.

*Treatment:*

Copyright © Mometrix Media. You have been licensed one copy of this document for personal use only. Any other reproduction or redistribution is strictly prohibited. All rights reserved.

- Supportive/symptomatic therapy.
- Dialysis and transplantation.

Uremic syndrome:

Uremic syndrome is a number of disorders that can occur with end-stage renal disease and renal failure, usually after multiple metabolic failures and decrease in creatinine clearance to <10 mL/min. There is compromise of all normal functions of the kidney: fluid balance, electrolyte balance, acid-base homeostasis, hormone production, and elimination of wastes. Metabolic abnormalities related to uremia include:

- **Decreased RBC production:** The kidney is unable to produce adequate erythropoietin in the peritubular cells, resulting in anemia, which is usually normocytic and normochromic. Parathyroid hormone levels may increase, causing calcification of the bone marrow, causing hypoproliferative anemia as RBC production is suppressed.
- **Platelet abnormalities:** ↓ Platelet count, increased turnover, and reduced adhesion leads to bleeding disorders.
- **Metabolic acidosis:** The tubular cells are unable to regulate acid-base metabolism, and phosphate, sulfuric, hippuric, and lactic acids increase, leading to congestive heart failure and weakness.
- **Hyperkalemia:** The nephron cannot excrete adequate amounts of potassium. Some drugs, such as diuretics that spare potassium may aggravate the condition.
- **Renal bone disease:** ↓ Calcium, ↑ phosphate, ↑ parathyroid hormone, and ↓ utilization of vitamin D lead to demineralization. In some cases, calcium and phosphate are deposited in other tissues (metastatic calcification).
- **Multiple endocrine disorders:** Thyroid hormone production is decreased and reproductive hormones abnormalities may result in infertility/impotence. Males have ↓ testosterone but ↑ estrogen and LH. Females experience irregular cycles, lack of ovulation, and menses. Insulin production may increase but with decreased clearance, resulting in episodes of hypoglycemia or decreased hyperglycemia in those who are diabetic.
- **Cardiovascular disorders:** Left ventricular hypertrophy is most common, but fluid retention may cause congestive heart failure, electrolyte imbalances, and dysrhythmias. Pericarditis, exacerbation of valvular disorders, and pericardial effusions may occur.
- **Anorexia and malnutrition:** Nausea and poor appetite contribute to hypoalbuminemia, sometimes exacerbated by restrictive diets.

## *Multisystem*
### Nosocomial infection

Nosocomial infection is defined by National Nosocomial Infections Surveillance (NNIS) as a hospital-acquired infection, either localized or systemic, caused by a pathogen or toxin that was not present (or incubating) in the patient at the time the patient entered the hospital. In some cases, infection may be obvious within the first 24-48 hours, but other infections may not be obvious until after discharge from the hospital because incubation times and resistance vary. An infection that occurs after discharge but is hospital-acquired is nosocomial. Identifying a nosocomial infection should result from analysis of laboratory findings as well as clinical symptoms. A diagnosis of infection by an attending physician or surgeon is also considered acceptable identification. Colonization that is not causing an inflammatory response or evidence of infection is not considered nosocomial for reporting purposes. The most common nosocomial infections are *Staphylococcus aureus* and Methicillin-resistant *Staphylococcus aureus (MRSA)*.

### *Clostridium difficile*

*Clostridium difficile* is an anaerobic Gram-positive bacillus that produces endospores. It is commonly found in healthcare facilities. Normal intestinal flora provide resistance to *C. difficile*, but if the flora is disrupted by antibiotic use (or sometimes chemotherapeutic agents) and the host is an asymptomatic carrier or has acquired

*Copyright © Mometrix Media. You have been licensed one copy of this document for personal use only. Any other reproduction or redistribution is strictly prohibited. All rights reserved.*

the infection during or after treatment, then *C. difficile* can begin to overgrow. *C. difficile* produces a lethal cytotoxin (Toxin B) and an endotoxin with cytotoxic action (Toxin A) that causes fluid to accumulate in the colon and causes severe damage to mucous membranes. *C. difficile* causes more nosocomial diarrhea cases than any other microorganism. All antibiotics can cause *C. difficile* infections but clindamycin and cephalosporins are most-frequently implicated. *Symptoms* vary widely, from mild diarrhea to lethal sepsis. *C. difficile* can cause diarrhea, colitis, and pseudomembranous colitis, and megacolon. Infection may not be obvious for weeks after completion of antibiotics. Spores are resistant to alcohol skin cleansers and to most soaps, so contact precautions with gloves should be used.

## Infectious diseases

VRE and MDRE:
Vancomycin-resistant *enterococci* (VRE) and multidrug-resistant *enterococci* (MDRE) have become severe cause for concern. VRE was first identified in the United States in 1989, but by 2004, it was the cause of one third of all hospital-acquired infections in intensive care units, related to the use of vancomycin. There are several phenotypes, but 2 types are common in the United States: Van A (resistant to vancomycin and teicoplanin) and Van B (resistant to just vancomycin). VRE infections are treatable by other antibiotics, but MDRE infections are increasingly resistant to 2 or more antibiotics, including vancomycin. Restriction of vancomycin use alone has not proven successful in controlling development of VRE or MDRE because other antibiotics, such as clindamycin, cephalosporin, aztreonam, ciprofloxacin, aminoglycoside, and metronidazole are implicated. Prior antibiotic use is present in almost all patients with MDRE. Precautions:
- Isolation with barrier precautions, gown and gloves during all patient contact, even entering the room.
- Hand hygiene both before and after contact and use of gloves.

- Dedicated equipment to reduce transmission.

## Tuberculosis

Tuberculosis (TB) **is** caused by *Mycobacterium tuberculosis*, an extracellular agent that needs oxygen and is attracted to the upper respiratory tract. It is also a facultative intracellular invader, allowing it to evade the immune system. The host immune system attempts to control the spread of *M. tuberculosis* by walling it off with macrophages, causing a positive skin reaction (cell-mediated immune response) but no infection. TB is a particular danger to those who are immunocompromised, with 8%-10% of those with HIV developing TB. Symptoms include weight loss, general debility, night sweats, fever, and (with pulmonary involvement) a progressive cough resulting in dyspnea and bloody sputum. Diagnosis is based on skin and sputum testing, as well as x-ray. Transmission is from suspended airborne particles, so anyone in contact with active TB is at risk of inhaling particles. Precautions:
- Prompt diagnosis and anti-tuberculosis drugs.
- Airborne infection isolation.
- Skin testing/x-rays of those in contact.
- Preventive Isoniazid therapy for those with latent infection or newly converted to positive on TB testing.

MDR-TB and XDR-TB:
Multidrug-resistant tuberculosis (MDR-TB) is resistant to at least 2 commonly used first-line drugs, isoniazid (INH) and rifampin, while extensively drug-resistant tuberculosis (XDR-TB) is also resistant to all fluoroquinolones and at least 1 of the 3 second-line drugs: amikacin, kanamycin, or capreomycin.
XDR-TB emerged as a worldwide concern in 2005. At present in the United States, XDR-TB is chiefly found in foreign born patients, but it also occurs in immunocompromised patients. Active TB requires treatment for extended periods of time, usually 18-24 months, with multiple drugs. Since the 1980s there has been an increased need to use second-line drugs to combat

*Copyright © Mometrix Media. You have been licensed one copy of this document for personal use only. Any other reproduction or redistribution is strictly prohibited. All rights reserved.*

infection. There are 2 primary causes for the increased resistance:

- Failure to complete a course of treatment.
- Mismanaged treatment, including incorrect medication, dosage, or duration of therapy.

People who have had previous TB are at increased risk and should be monitored carefully. Drug-resistant TB increasingly poses a risk for patients and staff in healthcare facilities.

Directly-observed therapy:
Adequate infection control for TB should include provisions for referring patients and/or staff with tuberculosis for directly-observed therapy (DOT) when indicated. DOT requires that a healthcare worker monitor every dose of an individual's anti-tuberculosis medication, ensuring that all medications are taken and the entire course of treatment is completed. Drug protocol may be changed to 2-3 times weekly rather than daily to facilitate DOT. Regulations about DOT vary from state to state. DOT is frequently used in these circumstances:

- Sputum cultures are positive for acid-fast bacilli.
- There is concurrent treatment with antiretroviral (HIV) drugs or methadone (for addiction).
- Infection is MDR-TB or XDR-TB.
- Co-morbidity with psychiatric disease or cognitive impairment exists.
- Patient is homeless and lacks adequate facilities.
- Patient has demonstrated lack of reliability in treatment.

When patients are discharged from the hospital, plans must include continuation of DOT through the use of home health agencies or having the patient return to a clinic for administration of drugs.

## Herpes zoster

Herpes zoster ("shingles") is caused by varicella zoster virus that is retained in the nerve cells after childhood chickenpox. The virus remains dormant until it is reactivated, often in older adults who are immunocompromised. Initial symptoms include pain (often severe burning) and redness. Painful blistering lesions then occur along sensory nerves usually in a line from the spine around to the chest although sometimes the head and face are involved. Facial nerve involvement can cause loss of taste and hearing. Eye involvement can cause blindness. The lesions eventually crust over and heal in 2-4 weeks, although some individuals have persistent post-herpetic neuralgia for 6-12 months. The lesions are contagious to those who contact them and have not been immunized or had chickenpox. The herpes zoster vaccine (single dose) is recommended for those ≥60 years of age to prevent shingles. *Treatment* for herpes includes analgesia (acetaminophen), acyclovir, Zostrix (capsaicin cream) to reduce the incidence of post-herpetic neuralgia, and rest.

## Hepatitis A

Hepatitis A is the cause of a serious liver disease, which can result in serious morbidity and death. Hepatitis A virus (HAV), an RNA picornavirus that replicates in the liver, is secreted into the gallbladder and enters the intestines. The virus triggers an antibody-mediated immune response with IgM that confers immunity, so reinfection and chronic infection do not occur. HAV infection is often asymptomatic in children, but adults may develop jaundice, general malaise, pain in the abdomen, nausea, and diarrhea. The virus is transmitted by the oral-fecal route, often from contamination on the hands or through sexual contact. On rare occasions, HAV has been transmitted in blood transfusions. Outbreaks have been traced to restaurants and kitchens in large facilities. Hepatitis A vaccine is now routinely given to children. Older adults may receive the 2-injection series if they are considered at risk, depending upon lifestyle (males having sex with other males or illegal drug users) or medical condition (chronic liver disease, those receiving clotting factor concentrates).

*Copyright © Mometrix Media. You have been licensed one copy of this document for personal use only.*
*Any other reproduction or redistribution is strictly prohibited. All rights reserved.*

## Hepatitis B

Hepatitis B virus (HBV) is a DNA virus of the family *Hepadnaviridae,* transmitted through contact with blood either directly, through sexual contact, or sharing needles. The DNA genome enters the host cell nucleus, copies, and replicates. The cell-mediated immune response that destroys the virus also causes damage to hepatic cells, resulting in acute hepatitis. Hepatitis B can cause serious liver disease leading to liver cancer. Because hepatitis B is transmitted through blood and body fluids, hepatitis B vaccine is now recommended for all newborns as well as all those<18 years of age and those in high-risk groups >18 years (drug users, men having sex with men, persons with multiple sex partners, partners of those with HBV, and healthcare workers). Older adults with end-stage renal disease (including those receiving hemodialysis), chronic liver disease, or HIV/AIDS should receive the vaccine.

## Hepatitis C

Hepatitis C virus (HCV) is a single-strand RNA *Flaviviridae* virus that binds to receptors on hepatic cells and enters to begin replicating. HCV readily mutates, which helps it to evade the host's immune response. There are 6 genotypes and several subtypes of HCV with some types more virulent and resistive to treatment than others. There is no vaccine. HCV is transmitted directly through blood or items, such as shared needles that are contaminated with blood. It can be spread by sexual contact. Prior to 1992, the blood supply was contaminated with HCV, as were clotting factors made before 1987. HCV causes an acute infection (first 6 months), but only about 20%-30% of individuals develop symptoms, such as fatigue, fever, jaundice, clay-colored stools, anorexia and fatigue; thus, many cases are undiagnosed. About 55%-85% go on to develop chronic infection, with 70% of those developing chronic liver disease. HCV is the primary reason for liver transplants.

## Scabies

Scabies is caused by a microscopic mite, *Sarcoptes scabiei hominis,* which tunnels under the outer layer of skin, raising small lines a few millimeters long. Mites prefer warm areas, such as between the fingers and in skin folds, but they can infest any area of the body. As the mites burrow, they cause intense itching and subsequent scratching can result in excoriation and secondary infections. Some individuals develop a generalized red rash. Scabies is spread very easily through person-to-person contact, and staff can easily spread infection among patients. Incubation time is 6-8 weeks, and itching usually begins in about 30 days, so people may be unaware they are transmitting scabies. Most infestations involve only about a dozen mites, but a severe form of scabies infection, Norwegian or crusted scabies, can occur in the elderly or those who are immunocompromised. This type usually causes less itching; however, the lesions can contain thousands of mites, making this type highly contagious. *Treatment* includes scabicides or oral medication (Ivermectin), antihistamines, and antibiotics for secondary infection.

## West Nile virus

West Nile virus (WNV) is an RNA virus, spread by infected mosquitoes. Infection has been traced to donor organs, blood transfusions, and breast milk although the blood supply has been monitored for WNV since 2003. While WNV is more common in adults, especially the elderly, it can affect infants and children, who show symptoms more readily than adults. The incubation period ranges from 2-14 days. There are 3 types of infection:

- *Viremia:* 80%, infection but no symptoms.
- *Mild:* 20% (West Nile fever), characterized by fever, malaise, lymphadenopathy, headache, rash, nausea, and vomiting. The acute stage usually is self-limiting to within a few days, but symptoms can persist for weeks. Symptoms include muscular weakness, fatigue, concentration problems,

*Copyright © Mometrix Media. You have been licensed one copy of this document for personal use only. Any other reproduction or redistribution is strictly prohibited. All rights reserved.*

fever, and headache. About 30% of infected individuals require hospitalization.

- *Severe*: <1%, severe neurological symptoms with meningitis and associated symptoms are the most common symptoms in children and young adults.

Treatment is supportive during illness and preventive (insect repellant).

## Human immunodeficiency virus

Human immunodeficiency virus (HIV) is a slow-acting retrovirus of the genus lentivirus. HIV binds with cells that have CD4 receptors, primarily CD4+ T cells and other cells of the immune system, enters the cells and begins replicating. Host cells are destroyed in a number of ways:

- Disruption of cell wall or cellular function may be caused after large numbers of replicated viral cells bud through the cell membrane or build up inside the cell.
- Formation of syncytia, occurring when cells infected with HIV fuse with nearby cells creating giant cells, thus, allowing HIV to spread from one cell to many.
- Apoptosis, or cell death, occurs when HIV sends a signal to uninfected cells, causing them to self-destruct.
- Binding to cell surface of uninfected cell by HIV gives the appearance that the cell is infected, causing it to be targeted by killer T cells as part of the immune response.
- HIV is spread through blood or other bodily fluids and blood-contaminated equipment.

## Acquired immunodeficiency syndrome

Acquired immunodeficiency syndrome (AIDS) is a progression of infection with human immunodeficiency virus (HIV). AIDS is diagnosed when the following criteria are met:

- HIV infection.
- CD4 count <200 cells/mm$^3$.
- AIDS defining condition, such as opportunistic infections (cytomegalovirus, tuberculosis), wasting syndrome, neoplasms

(Kaposi's sarcoma), or AIDS dementia complex.

Because there is such a wide range of AIDS defining conditions, the patient may present with many types of *symptoms*, depending upon the diagnosis, but more than half of AIDS patients exhibit fever, lymphadenopathy, pharyngitis, rash, and myalgia/arthralgia. It is important to review the following:

- CD4 counts, to determine immune status.
- WBC and differential for signs of infection.
- Cultures to help identify any infective agents.
- Complete blood count to evaluate for signs of bleeding or thrombocytopenia.

*Treatment* aims to cure or manage opportunistic conditions and control underlying HIV infection through highly active anti-retroviral therapy (HAART), 3 or more drugs used concurrently.

Antiretroviral agents:
There are 4 primary classes of antiretroviral agents used for the treatment of HIV/AIDS:

- *Non-nucleoside reverse transcriptase inhibitors* (NNRTIs), such as delavirdine (Rescriptor®), efavirenz (Sustiva®), and Nevirapine (Viramune®) bind to reverse transcriptase and disable it. Reverse transcriptase is a protein required for HIV replication.
- *Nucleoside reverse transcriptase inhibitors* (NRTIs), such as abacavir (Ziagen®), abacavir + lamivudine (Epzicom®), zidovudine (AZT®), and lamivudine (Epivir®) are defective versions of building blocks necessary for replication. When HIV binds to the defective version, it is unable to complete replication.
- *Protease inhibitors* (PIs) disable the protein protease, which HIV requires in order to replicate. PIs include amprenavir (Agenerase®), indinavir (Crixivan®), and nelfinavir (Viracept®).
- *Fusion inhibitors,* such as enfuvirtide (Fuzeon®) are entry blockers.

*Copyright © Mometrix Media. You have been licensed one copy of this document for personal use only. Any other reproduction or redistribution is strictly prohibited. All rights reserved.*

## Toxic shock syndrome

Toxic shock syndrome (TSS) is an acute severe life-threatening bacterial infection that causes a systemic infection with high fever, hypotension, myalgia, diarrhea and widespread erythematous rash that has the appearance of bad sunburn, with subsequent desquamation (peeling). The original causative agent was *Staphylococcus aureus*, and infections were related to use of tampons, but the infection can occur with wounds or surgical sites where the bacteria can find entry. There are now 2 forms: *Staphylococcus aureus* (TSS) and *Streptococcal toxic shock syndrome* (STSS). *STSS* occurs secondary to an infection in the body, often an infected wound, causing severe hypotension, dyspnea, tachycardia, liver and kidney failure, and a splotchy rash that may peel. Treatment includes:

- Hospitalization with aggressive antibiotic therapy.
- Intravenous fluids to treat hypotension.
- Topical non-adhesive, non-occlusive dressings with absorbent materials, as indicated.

## Necrotizing fasciitis

Necrotizing fasciitis is a rapidly spreading infection of the soft tissues involving extensive necrosis of the fascia and subcutaneous tissue as well as destruction of the vasculature resulting from thrombosis. It most often occurs in the extremities after a minor infection. The most common organisms are group A β-hemolytic *Streptococci* but there may be polymicrobial infections or other causative agents. It may result from surgical procedures, including cardiac catheterization. The infection begins with pain, edema, fever, toxemia, and cellulitis that spreads rapidly, becoming increasingly cyanotic as tissue and perfusion is impaired. Bullae form and progress to necrosis and gangrene and sepsis within 3-5 days. The mortality rate is 25%. *Treatment* includes:

- Aggressive extensive surgical debridement of all non-viable tissue. Repeat surgical debridement may be necessary.

- Antibiotic therapy.
- Wound care as indicated by the extent of the wound with careful monitoring to determine if wound is deteriorating.
- IV immunoglobulin may be used.

## Topical antibiotics

Topical antibiotics may be used to treat localized wound infections based on results of culture and sensitivities so that the treatment is appropriate for the invading microorganism. Topical antibiotics include:

- ***Cadexomer iodine*** (Iodosorb®) is an iodine preparation formulated to be less toxic to granulating tissue. It is applied as powder, paste, or ointment. The ointment contains beads with iodine. The beads swell in contact with exudate, slowly releasing the iodine, which is effective against a broad range of bacteria, *Staphylococcus aureus, MRSA, Streptococcus, and Pseudomonas,* as well as viruses and fungi.
- ***Gentamicin sulphate,*** prepared as a cream or ointment, is a broad-spectrum antibiotic that is effective against both primary and secondary skin infections in stasis and other ulcers or skin lesions. It is bacteriocidal against *Staphylococcus aureus, Streptococcus, and Pseudomonas,* but it does not have antiviral or antifungal properties.
- ***Metronidazole,*** prepared as a gel or a wax-glycerin cream, is effective against MRSA infections.
- ***Mupirocin*** *2%,* prepared in an ointment, is effective primarily against Gram-positive bacteria and is used primarily for *Staphylococcus, MRSA,* and *Streptococcus.* It is frequently used to treat nasal colonization of *Staphylococcus* because colonization is implicated in subsequent wound infections.
- ***Polymyxin B sulphate-Bacitracin zinc-neomycin ointment*** (Neosporin®) is frequently used to prevent infections in small cuts and lacerations, but it can also be used in infected wounds and is active against *Staphylococcus aureus, Streptococcus and Pseudomonas.*

*Copyright © Mometrix Media. You have been licensed one copy of this document for personal use only. Any other reproduction or redistribution is strictly prohibited. All rights reserved.*

- **Polymyxin B sulphate-Gramicidin cream** is similar to the preceding item except it is also effective against *MRSA*.
- **Silver sulfadiazine** (2%-7%) is frequently used in burn treatment and has a strong antimicrobial action against *Staphylococcus aureus, MRSA, Streptococcus, and Pseudomonas.*
- **Silver (ionized),** prepared in absorbent sheets and activated with sterile water, is effective against the same organisms as silver sulfadiazine. The moist environment increases reepithelialization.

## Fistulas

Classification systems for fistulas help to characterize the fistula and assist in the management and treatment. Sometimes, more than one classification may be used. For example, a fistula may be described as "Complex, Type I with small to medium output."
- **Simple—Complex:** This system classifies fistulas according to involvement:
  - o *Simple* fistulas are short and have direct tracts with no organ involvement or abscess.
  - o *Complex, Type I* involves multiple organs, and there is an abscess associated with the fistula.
  - o *Complex, Type II* has a fistula opening into the base of a disrupted wound.
- **Volume:** With this classification system, the fistula is classified according to the amount of drainage from the wound in a 24-hour period.
  - o *Low-output* fistulas drain less than 150 ml per 24 hours.
  - o *Small to medium output* fistulas drain 150-500 ml per 24 hours.
  - o *High output* fistulas drain more than 500 ml per 24 hours.

Protecting skin:
Providing skin protection for draining wounds, such as fistulas, is critical. Low output fistulas may need only skin barriers and easily-changed absorbent dressings. Creases, folds, and depressions may need to be filled with skin barrier paste, wafers, or powder before solid barriers are applied. *Solid barriers* last as long as they remain intact; *liquid skin sealants,* up to 24 hours; and *skin powders/pastes,* up to 24 hours. Containing drainage is necessary. If drainage cannot be contained with an absorbent dressing, then ostomy appliances with solid skin barriers and pouches are indicated. The barrier should extend at least 1.5 inches around the perimeter of the fistula. The barrier must adhere to skin to avoid drainage getting under the barrier, so the opening may need to be enlarged. Pouching systems with barriers that can be cut to fit usually work best. If the drainage is extensive, a bedside drainage bag may be used. Very large wounds (more than 4 inches) may require a custom pouching system.

Treatments:
Fistula treatment includes:
- **Antibiotics:** Antibiotics, such as metronidazole, are the first line of treatment but are often combined with other therapies, such as surgical drainage or excision.
- **Corticosteroids**: Corticosteroids may be used in conjunction with antibiotics and other therapy for Crohn's disease.
- **Drains**: There is evidence that treating abscesses with antibiotics and drainage can prevent fistula formation. Drains/tubes may be left in place to ensure drainage or keep existing fistulas open.
- **Seton**: A suture is placed to hold the fistula open (draining seton). If a fistula heals at the surface and remains open underneath, the discharge will tunnel to the surface again.
- **Autologous fibrin glue:** Glue is used to close the fistula.
- **Fistulotomy/Fistulectomy:** Excision is often the most effective treatment for a fistula. Staged repairs may be done. Surgical treatment may involve open surgery, endoscopic, or laparoscopic approaches. Conservative treatment may precede surgical therapy, but terminal or Crohn's disease patients are poor surgical candidates.

*Copyright © Mometrix Media. You have been licensed one copy of this document for personal use only. Any other reproduction or redistribution is strictly prohibited. All rights reserved.*

## Drains

Simple drains are latex or vinyl tubes of varying sizes and lengths inserted into a wound to provide drainage of serous material, blood, pus, or other discharge. This type of drain is usually placed through a stab wound near the area of involvement.

Penrose drains are soft rubber/latex tubes that are flat in appearance and are placed in surgical wounds to drain fluid by gravity and capillary action. They are available in various diameters and lengths.

Sump drains are double-lumen or tri-lumen tubes (with a third lumen for infusions). A large outflow lumen and small inflow lumen produces venting when air enters the inflow lumen and forces drainage into the large lumen.

Percutaneous drainage catheter is inserted into the wound to provide continuous drainage for the infection or for collection of drainage in the wound. Irrigation of the catheter may need to be done to maintain patency. Skin barriers and pouching systems may be necessary.

Closed wound drainage systems:
Closed drainage systems use low-pressure suction to provide continuous gravity drainage of wounds. Drains are attached to collapsible suction reservoirs that provide negative pressure. *Management* includes daily dressing changes about the tube insertion site, inspection of skin for inflammation or drainage, monitoring type and amount of drainage from the device, and emptying the device by holding it lower than the wound, opening the plug, draining, squeezing all air out to reestablish suction and negative pressure, and reinserting the plug. There are 2 closed drainage systems that are in frequent use: Jackson-Pratt® and Hemovac®.
- **Jackson-Pratt®** is a bulb-type drain that is about the size of a lemon. A thin plastic drain from the wound extends to a squeeze bulb that can hold about 100 ml of drainage.
- **Hemovac®** is a round drain with coiled springs inside that are compressed after emptying to create suction. The device can hold up to 500 ml of drainage.

## Wound therapy

Negative pressure wound therapy (NPWT) uses subatmospheric (negative) pressure with a suction unit and a semi-occlusive vapor-permeable dressing. The suction reduces periwound and interstitial edema, decompressing vessels and improving circulation. It also stimulates the production of new cells and decreases the colonization of bacteria. NPWT also increases the rate of granulation and re-epithelialization so that wounds heal more quickly. The wound must be debrided of necrotic tissue prior to treatment. NPWT is used for a variety of difficult to heal wounds, especially those that show less than 30% healing in 4 weeks of post-debridement treatment or those with excessive exudate:
- Chronic stage II and IV pressure ulcers.
- Skin flaps.
- Diabetic ulcers.
- Acute wounds.
- Burns, both partial and full-thickness.
- Unresponsive arterial and venous ulcers.
- Surgical wounds and those with dehiscence.

It is contraindicated in some conditions: wound malignancy, untreated osteomyelitis, exposed blood vessels or organs, and nonenteric, unexplored fistulas.

*Application:* Application of negative pressure wound therapy is done after the wound is determined to be appropriate for this treatment and debridement is completed, leaving the wound tissue exposed. There are a number of different electrical suction NPWT systems, such as the VAC® (vacuum-assisted closure) system and the Versatile I® (VI). Application steps include:
- Apply nonadherent porous foam cut to fit and completely cover the wound.
  - Polyurethane (hydrophobic, repelling moisture) is used for all wounds EXCEPT those that are painful, have tunneling or sinus tracts, deep trauma wounds, and

*Copyright © Mometrix Media. You have been licensed one copy of this document for personal use only. Any other reproduction or redistribution is strictly prohibited. All rights reserved.*

wounds needing controlled growth of granulation.
  o Polyvinyl (hydrophilic) is used for all wounds EXCEPT deep wounds with moderate granulation, deep pressure ulcers, and flaps.
- Secure foam occlusive transparent film.
- Cut opening to accommodate the drainage tube in the dressing and attach drainage tube.
- Attach tube to suction canister, creating closed system.
- Set pressure to 75-125, as indicated.
- Change dressings 2-3 times weekly.

## WBC count

White blood cell (leukocyte) count is used as an indicator of bacterial and viral infection. WBC is reported as the total number of all white blood cells.
Normal WBC for adults:  4,800-10,000
Acute infection:  10,000+
Severe infection:  30,000
Viral infection: 4,000 and below

The differential provides the percentage of each different type of leukocyte. An increase in the white blood cell count is usually related to an increase in one type and often an increase in immature neutrophils, known as bands, referred to as a "shift to the left, an indication of an infectious process:

| Immature neutrophils (bands) | 1%-3% | Increase with infection. |
|---|---|---|
| Segmented neutrophils (Segs) | 50%-62% | Increase with acute, localized, or systemic bacterial infections. |
| Eosinophils | 0-3% | Decrease with stress and acute infection. |
| Basophils | 0-1% | Decrease during acute stage of infection. |
| Lymphocytes | 25%-40% | Increase in some viral and bacterial infections. |
| Monocytes | 3%-7% | Increase during recovery stage of |

| | | acute infection. |
|---|---|---|

## Antibiotic classification

Antibiotics may be classified according to their chemical nature, origin, action, or range of effectiveness. There are hundreds of antibiotics. Broad-spectrum antibiotics are useful against both Gram-positive and Gram-negative bacteria. Medium spectrum antibiotics are usually effective against Gram-positive bacteria, although some may be effective against Gram-negative bacteria, as well. Narrow spectrum antibiotics are effective against a small range of bacteria. Antibiotics function by killing the bacteria by interfering with its biological functions (bacteriocidal) or by preventing reproduction (bacteriostatic). The main classes of antibiotics include:

- **Macrolides:**  Medium spectrum antibiotics. They prevent protein production by bacteria and are primarily bacteriostatic but may be bactericidal at high doses. They may be irritating to the gastric mucosa, but they are less likely to cause allergic responses than penicillins or cephalosporins. Macrolides include erythromycin (E-Mycin®), clarithromycin (Biaxin®), and azithromycin (Zithromax®).
- **Penicillins:**  Medium spectrum antibiotics may be combined with β-lactamase inhibitors. They are bacteriocidal and cause breakdown of the bacterial cell wall. They may cause severe allergic reactions in sensitive individuals. Penicillins include penicillin, ampicillin, and amoxicillin.
- **Cephalosporins:**  Medium spectrum antibiotics effective against Gram-negative organisms. They are bacteriocidal and inhibit cell wall synthesis. They are divided into different "generations" according to antimicrobial properties, with succeeding generations having more powerful effects against resistant strains. First generation includes cephazolin (Kefzol®), cephalexin (Keflex®), and cephradine (Velosef®). Second generation includes cefaclor (Ceclor®), cefuroxime (Zinacef®), and loracarbef (Lorabid®). Third generation includes

Copyright © Mometrix Media. You have been licensed one copy of this document for personal use only. Any other reproduction or redistribution is strictly prohibited. All rights reserved.

cefotaxime (Claforan®), cefixime (Suprax®), cefpodoxime (Vantin®), ceftazidime (Fortax®), and cefdinir (Omnicef®). A fourth generation antibiotic is cefepime (Maxipime®).

- **Polymyxins:** Narrow spectrum antibiotics effective against Gram-negative organisms. They interfere with the cell membrane of bacteria and are bactericidal. Polymyxins have both neurotoxic and nephrotoxic properties and are not used unless other antibiotics are ineffective. They must be given intravenously. A drug in this group is Polymyxin B Sulfate®.
- **Fluoroquinolones:** Broad-spectrum antibiotics that inhibit bacterial reproduction and repair of genetic material in the bacterial DNA. Drugs include ciprofloxacin (Cipro®), levofloxacin (Levaquin®), and ofloxacin (Floxin®).
- **Sulfonamides:** Sulfonamides are medium-spectrum antibiotics with action against Gram-positive and many Gram-negative organisms, as well as *Plasmodium* and *Toxoplasma*. Some people sensitive to these antibiotics may develop an allergic response. Resistance to sulfa drugs is widespread. Sulfa drugs interfere with folate synthesis and prevent cell division, so they are bacteriostatic. Sulfonamides include co-trimoxazole (Bactrim®) and trimethoprim (Proloprim®).
- **Tetracyclines:** Broad-spectrum antibiotics. They are also used for rickettsiae and psittacosis-producing agents. Tetracyclines include tetracycline, doxycycline (Vibramycin®), and minocycline.
- **Aminoglycosides:** Effective against Gram-negative bacteria. They interfere with protein production in the bacteria and are bacteriocidal. Aminoglycosides cannot be taken orally. They are often given in conjunction with other classes of antibiotics, such as penicillin. Aminoglycosides include gentamicin (Garamycin®) and tobramycin (Tobrex®), neomycin, and streptomycin.

## Shock

There are a number of different types of shock, but there are general characteristics that they have in common. In all types of shock, there is a marked decrease in tissue perfusion related to hypotension, so that there is insufficient oxygen delivered to the tissues and, in turn, inadequate removal of cellular waste products, causing injury to tissue:

- Hypotension (systolic <90 mm Hg). BP may be somewhat higher (110 mm Hg) in those who are initially hypertensive.
- Tachycardia (>90 bpm).
- Bradypnea (<7 breaths per minute) or tachypnea (>29 breaths per minute). This varies depending upon the cause of the shock.
- Decreased urinary output (<0.5 mL/kg/hr), especially marked in hypovolemic shock.
- Metabolic acidosis.
- Hypoxemia (<90 mm Hg for children and persons up to 50 years of age, <80 mm Hg for those 51 to 70, and <70 mm Hg for those over 70.
- Peripheral/cutaneous vasoconstriction/vasodilation.
- Alterations in mental status with dullness, agitation, anxiety, or lethargy.

Distributive shock:
Distributive shock occurs when there is adequate blood volume but inadequate intravascular volume because of arterial/venous dilation that results in decreased vascular tone and hypoperfusion of internal organs. Cardiac output may be normal or blood may pool, decreasing cardiac output. Distributive shock may result from anaphylactic shock, septic shock, neurogenic shock, and drug ingestions.
*Symptoms*:
- Hypotension (systolic <90 mm Hg or <40 mm Hg change from normal), tachypnea, tachycardia (>90 bpm) (may be lower if patient receiving β-blockers.
- Skin initially warm, later hypoperfused.
- Hyper- or hypothermia (>38ºC or <36ºC).
- Hypoxemia. Alterations in mentation.

*Copyright © Mometrix Media. You have been licensed one copy of this document for personal use only. Any other reproduction or redistribution is strictly prohibited. All rights reserved.*

- Urinary output. Symptoms related to underlying cause.

*Diagnostic* procedures are similar to those for septic and anaphylactic shock.

*Treatment* includes treating the underlying cause and stabilizing the hemodynamics:
- Septic or anaphylactic therapy and monitoring as indicated.
- Oxygen with endotracheal intubation, if necessary.
- Rapid fluid administration at 0.25-0.5L NS or isotonic crystalloid every 5-10 minutes as needed to 2-3 L. (Children: 5-10 mL/kg to 30 mL/kg maximum).
- Inotropes (dopamine, dobutamine, norepinephrine), if necessary.

Neurogenic shock:
Neurogenic shock occurs when injury to the CNS (from trauma resulting in acute spinal cord injury (from both blunt and penetrating injuries), neurological diseases, drugs, or anesthesia, impairs the autonomic nervous system that controls the cardiovascular system. *Symptoms* include hypotension and warm dry skin (related to lack of vascular tone) that becomes hypothermia from loss of cutaneous heat. Bradycardia is a common but not universal symptom. The degree of symptoms relates to the level of injury with injuries above T1 capable of causing disruption of the entire sympathetic nervous system and lower injuries causing various degrees of disruption. Even incomplete spinal cord injury can cause neurogenic shock. *Treatment* includes:
- ABCDE (airway, breathing, circulation, disability evaluation, exposure)
- Rapid fluid administration with crystalloid to keep mean arterial pressure at 85-90 mm Hg.
- Placement of pulmonary artery catheter to monitor fluid overload.
- Inotropes (dopamine, dobutamine) if fluids don't correct hypotension.
- Atropine for persistent bradycardia.
- Transfer to trauma unit or facility.

Hypovolemic shock:
Hypovolemic shock occurs when there is inadequate intravascular fluid:
- The loss may be *absolute* because of an internal shifting of fluid or an external loss of fluid, as occurs with massive hemorrhage, thermal injuries, severe vomiting or diarrhea, and injuries (such as ruptured spleen or dissecting arteries) that interfere with intravascular integrity.
- Hypovolemia may also be *relative* and related to vasodilation, increased capillary membrane permeability from sepsis or injuries, and decreased colloidal osmotic pressure that may occur with loss of sodium and some disorders, such as hypopituitarism and cirrhosis.

Hypovolemic shock is classified according to the degree of fluid loss:
- *Class I:* <750 mL or ≤15% of total circulating volume (TCV). Heart rate (HR) <100 bpm, BP normal.
- *Class II:* 750-100 mL or 15%-30% of TCV. HR >100 bpm, BP normal.
- *Class III:* 1500-2000 mL or 30%-40% of TCV. HR >120 bpm, BP decreased.
- *Class IV:* >2000 mL or >40% of TCV. HR >140 bpm, BP decreased.

**Anaphylaxis syndrome**

Anaphylaxis syndrome is a sudden acute systemic immunoglobulin E (IgE) or non-immunoglobulin E (non-IgE) inflammatory response affecting the cardiopulmonary and other systems.
- *IgE-mediated response* (anaphylactic shock) is an antibody-antigen reaction against an allergen, such as milk, peanuts, latex, insect bites, or fish. This is the most common type.
- *Non IgE-mediated response* (anaphylactoid reaction) is a systemic reaction to infection, exercise, radio contrast material or other triggers. While the response is almost identical to the other type, it does not involve IgE.

Copyright © Mometrix Media. You have been licensed one copy of this document for personal use only. Any other reproduction or redistribution is strictly prohibited. All rights reserved.

Typically, with IgE-mediated response, an antigen triggers release of substances, such as histamine and prostaglandins, which affect the skin, cardiopulmonary, and GI systems. Histamine causes initial erythema and edema by inducing vasodilation. Each time the person has contact with the antigen, more antibodies form in response, so allergic reactions worsen with each contact. In some cases, initial reactions may be mild, but subsequent contact can cause severe, life-threatening response.

Symptoms and treatment:
Anaphylaxis syndrome may present with a few symptoms or a wide range that encompasses cardiopulmonary, dermatological, and gastrointestinal responses. *Symptoms* may recur after the initial treatment (biphasic anaphylaxis), so careful monitoring is essential:

- Sudden onset of weakness, dizziness, confusion.
- Severe generalized edema and angioedema. Lips and tongue may swell.
- Urticaria.
- Increased permeability of vascular system and loss of vascular tone.
- Severe hypotension leading to shock.
- Laryngospasm/bronchospasm with obstruction of airway causing dyspnea and wheezing.
- Nausea, vomiting, and diarrhea.
- Seizures, coma and death.

*Treatment* includes
- Establish patent airway and intubate if necessary for ventilation.
- Provide oxygen at 100% high flow.
- Monitor VS.
- Epinephrine (Epi-pen® or 1:1000 solution to 0.1 mg/kg/wt).
- 2.5 mg albuterol per nebulizer for bronchospasm.
- Intravenous fluids to provide bolus of fluids for hypotension.
- Diphenhydramine 1.0 mg/kg/wt (to 25 mg) if shock persists.
- Methylprednisolone 2.0 mg/kg/wt if no response to other drugs.

## Severe infections

There are a number of terms used to refer to severe infections and often used interchangeably, but they are part of a continuum:

- **Bacteremia** is the presence of bacteria in the blood but without systemic infection.
- **Septicemia** is a systemic infection caused by pathogens (usually bacteria or fungi) present in the blood.
- **Systemic inflammatory response syndrome** *(SIRS)*, a generalized inflammatory response affecting many organ systems, may be caused by infectious or non-infectious agents, such as trauma, burns, adrenal insufficiency, pulmonary embolism, and drug overdose. If an infectious agent is identified or suspected, SIRS is an aspect of sepsis. Infectious agents include a wide range of bacteria and fungi, including *Streptococcus pneumoniae* and *Staphylococcus aureus*. SIRS includes 2 of the following:
  o Elevated (>38°C) or subnormal rectal temperature (<36°C).
  o Tachypnea or $PaCO_2$ <32 mm Hg.
  o Tachycardia.
  o Leukocytosis (>12,000) or leukopenia (<4000).

Infections can progress from bacteremia, septicemia, and SIRS to the following:

- **Sepsis** is the presence of infection, either locally or systemically, in which there is a generalized life-threatening inflammatory response (SIRS). It includes all the indications for SIRS as well as one of the following:
  o Changes in mental status.
  o Hypoxemia (<72 mm Hg) without pulmonary disease.
  o Elevation in plasma lactate.
  o Decreased urinary output <5 mL/kg/wt for ≥1 hour.
- **Severe sepsis** includes both indications of SIRS and sepsis as well as indications of increasing organ dysfunction with inadequate perfusion and/or hypotension.

*Copyright © Mometrix Media. You have been licensed one copy of this document for personal use only.*
*Any other reproduction or redistribution is strictly prohibited. All rights reserved.*

- **Septic shock** is a progression from severe sepsis. In septic shock, refractory hypotension occurs despite treatment. There may be indications of lactic acidosis.
- **Multi-organ dysfunction syndrome (MODS)** is the most common cause of sepsis-related death. Cardiac function becomes depressed, acute respiratory distress syndrome (ARDS) may develop, and renal failure may follow an acute tubular necrosis or cortical necrosis. Thrombocytopenia appears in about 30% of those affected and may result in disseminated intravascular coagulation (DIC). Liver damage and bowel necrosis may occur.

Multi-organ dysfunction syndrome

Multi-organ dysfunction syndrome is progressive deterioration and failure of 2 or more organ systems with mortality rates of 45%-50% if 2 organ systems are involved and up to 80%-100% if there are ≥3 systems failing. Trauma patients and those with severe conditions, such as shock, burns, and sepsis, are particularly vulnerable, especially patients >65 years of age. MODS may be primary or secondary:

- **Primary** MODS refers to direct injury/disorder of the organ systems, resulting in dysfunction, such as with thermal injuries, traumatic pulmonary injuries, and invasive infections.
- **Secondary** MODS refers to dysfunction of organ systems not directly involved in injury/disorder but developing as the result of a systemic inflammatory response syndrome (SIRS) as the coordination between the patient's immune and inflammatory responses fails. In some patients, failure of organ systems is sequential, usually progressing from the lungs, the liver, the gastrointestinal system, and the kidneys to the heart. However, in other cases, various organ systems may fail at the same time.

## Septic shock

Septic shock is caused by toxins produced by bacteria and cytokines that the body produces in response to severe infection, resulting in a complex syndrome of disorders. *Symptoms* are wide-ranging:

- Initial: Hyper- or hypothermia, ↑ temperature (↑ 38ºC) with chills, tachycardia with ↑ pulse pressure, tachypnea, alterations in mental status (dullness), hypotension, hyperventilation with respiratory alkalosis (PaCO$_2$ ≤30 mm Hg), ↑ lactic acid, and unstable BP, and dehydration with ↑ urinary output.
- Cardiovascular: Myocardial depression and dysrhythmias.
- Respiratory: Adults respiratory distress syndrome (ARDS).
- Renal: acute renal failure (ARF) with ↓ urinary output and ↑ BUN.
- Hepatic: Jaundice and liver dysfunction with ↑ in transaminase, alkaline phosphatase and bilirubin.
- Hematologic: Mild or severe blood loss (from mucosal ulcerations), neutropenia or neutrophilia, ↓ platelets, and DIC.
- Endocrine: Hyperglycemia, hypoglycemia (rare).
- Skin: cellulitis, erysipelas, and fasciitis; acrocyanotic and necrotic peripheral lesions.

Diagnosis and treatment:
Septic shock is apt to occur in newborns, adults who are >50 years of age, and those who are immunocompromised. There is no specific test to confirm a diagnosis of septic shock, so the diagnosis is based on clinical findings and tests that evaluate hematologic, infectious, and metabolic states: CBC, DIC panel, electrolytes, liver function tests, BUN, creatinine, blood glucose, ABGs, urinalysis, ECG, radiographs, and blood and urine cultures. *Treatment* must be aggressive and includes:
- Oxygen and endotracheal intubation, as necessary.
- IV access with 2-large bore catheters and a central venous line.

*Copyright © Mometrix Media. You have been licensed one copy of this document for personal use only. Any other reproduction or redistribution is strictly prohibited. All rights reserved.*

- Rapid fluid administration at 0.5 L NS or isotonic crystalloid every 5-10 minutes, as needed (to 4-6 L); (Children: 10 mL/kg to total 60 mL/kg).
- Monitoring urinary output to optimal >30 mL/hr (1 mL/hr for children).
- Inotropes (dopamine, dobutamine, norepinephrine), if no response to fluids or fluid overload.
- Empiric IV antibiotic therapy (usually with 2 broad spectrum antibiotics for both gram-positive and gram-negative bacteria) until cultures return and antibiotics may be changed.
- Hemodynamic and laboratory monitoring.
- Removing source of infection (abscess, catheter).

## Behavioral

### Delirium

Delirium is an acute sudden change in consciousness, characterized by a reduced ability to focus or sustain attention, language and memory disturbance, disorientation, confusion, audiovisual hallucinations, sleep disturbance, and psychomotor activity disorder. Delirium differs from disorders with similar symptoms in that delirium is fluctuating. Delirium occurs in 10%-40% of hospitalized older adults and about 80% of patients who are terminally ill. Delirium may result from drugs, such as anticholinergics, and from numerous conditions, including infection, hypoxia, trauma, dementia, depression, vision and hearing loss, surgery, alcoholism, untreated pain, fluid/electrolyte imbalance, and malnutrition. Delirium increases the risk of morbidity and death, especially if untreated. *Diagnosis* includes conducting an interview to identify triggers, obtaining a history, and reviewing the chart. Simple tasks, such as asking the patient to count backward from 20 to 1 and to spell her first name backward, can be used to identify attention deficit. *Treatment* includes providing a caretaker or sitter to ensure personal safety and decreasing the dosage of any hypnotics and psychotropics. Medications that have been found to reduce symptoms include trazodone, lorazepam, and haloperidol.

Confusion Assessment Method:
The Confusion Assessment Method is used to assess the development of delirium and is intended for use by those without psychiatric training. The tool covers 9 factors. Some factors have a range of possibilities, and others are rated only as to whether the characteristic is present, not present, whether uncertainty exists, or the characteristic is not applicable. The tool provides room to describe abnormal behavior. Factors indicative of delirium include:

- *Onset*: Acute change in mental status.
- *Attention*: Inattentive, stable, or fluctuating.
- *Thinking*: Disorganized, rambling conversation, switching topics, illogical.
- *Level of consciousness:* Altered, ranging from alert to coma.
- *Orientation*: Disoriented (regarding person, place, time).
- *Memory*: Impaired.
- *Perceptual disturbances:* Hallucinations, illusions.
- *Psychomotor abnormalities:* Agitation (tapping, picking, moving) or retardation (staring, not moving).
- *Sleep-wake cycle:* Awake at night and sleepy in the daytime.

The Confusion Assessment tool indicates delirium if there is an acute onset with fluctuating inattention and disorganized thinking or altered level of consciousness.

### Non-Alzheimer's dementias

Non-Alzheimer's dementia includes:
- *Creutzfeldt-Jakob disease:* This causes rapidly progressive dementia with impaired memory, behavioral changes, and incoordination.
- *Dementia with Lewy Bodies:* Cognitive and physical decline is similar to Alzheimer's, but symptoms may fluctuate frequently. This form of dementia may include visual hallucinations, muscle rigidity, and tremors.

*Copyright © Mometrix Media. You have been licensed one copy of this document for personal use only. Any other reproduction or redistribution is strictly prohibited. All rights reserved.*

- **Fronto-temporal dementia:** This may cause marked changes in personality and behavior and is characterized by difficulty using and understanding language.
- **Mixed dementia:** Dementia mirrors Alzheimer's and another type because there are two different causes of dementia.
- **Normal pressure hydrocephalus:** This is characterized by ataxia, memory loss, and urinary incontinence.
- **Parkinson's dementia:** This form of dementia may involve impaired decision making as well as difficulty concentrating, learning new material, understanding complex language, and sequencing.
- Inflexibility is observed. Short or long-term memory loss may occur.
- **Vascular dementia:** Memory loss may be less pronounced than that observed with Alzheimer's, but the symptoms are similar.

## Alzheimer's disease

There are a number of methods for staging Alzheimer's disease. Staging is done by a combination of physical exam, history (often provided by family or caregivers), and mental assessment, as there is no definitive test for Alzheimer's. The 7-stage classification system that was developed by Gary Reisberg, MD is used by the Alzheimer's Association.

Staging of Alzheimer's disease:

| | |
|---|---|
| **Stage 1** | Pre-clinical with no evident impairment although slight changes may be occurring within the brain. |
| **Stage 2** | Very mild cognitive decline with some misplacing of items and forgetting things or words, but impairment is not usually noticeable to others or found on medical examination. |
| **Stage 3** | Mild, early-stage cognitive decline with short-term memory loss, problems with reading retention, remembering names, handling money, planning, and organizing. May misplace items of value. |

| | |
|---|---|
| **Stage 4** | Moderate cognitive decline with decreased knowledge of current affairs or family history, difficulty doing complex tasks, and social withdrawal. This stage is more easily recognized on exam and may persist for 2-10 years, during which the patients may be able to manage most activities of daily living and hygiene. |
| **Stage 5** | Moderately-severe cognitive decline as the cerebral cortex and hippocampus shrink and the ventricles enlarge. Patients are obviously confused and disoriented regarding date, time, and place. Patients may have difficulty using/understanding speech and managing the activities of daily living. They may forget their address and telephone number. They may dress inappropriately, forget to eat and lose weight, or eat a poor diet. They may be unable to do simple math, such as counting backward by 2s. |
| **Stage 6** | Moderately severe cognitive decline as the brain continues to shrink and neurons die. Patients are profoundly confused and unable to care for themselves and may undergo profound personality changes. They may confuse fiction and reality. They may fail to recognize family members, experience difficulty toileting, and begin to pace obsessively or wander away. Sundowner's syndrome, in which the person has disruption of waking/sleeping cycles and tends to get restless and wander about at night, is common. Patients may develop obsessive behaviors, such as tearing items, pulling at their hair, or wringing their hands. This stage (with stage 7) may be prolonged, lasting 1-5 years. |

*Copyright © Mometrix Media. You have been licensed one copy of this document for personal use only. Any other reproduction or redistribution is strictly prohibited. All rights reserved.*

| Stage 7 | Very severe cognitive decline during which most patients are wheelchair bound or bedbound and lose most ability to speak beyond a few words. They are incontinent of urine and feces, and they may be unable to sit unsupported or hold their head up. They choke easily and have increased weakness and rigidity of muscles. |
|---|---|

Treatment:

Treatment for Alzheimer's disease is aimed at slowing the progression of the disease and ensuring patient safety. Two types of drugs are FDA approved, but many clinical trials are still taking place. In some cases, 2 drugs (such as Aricept® and Namenda®) may be given. Patients must take medication daily and be monitored carefully because some drugs may worsen symptoms in some patients, so different drugs may need to be tried.

| Type of Drug | Type of drug and indication | Adverse effects |
|---|---|---|
| **Cholin-esterase inhibitor** (Prevents breakdown of acetylcholine, needed for learning and memory) | Donepezil (Aricept®): All stages of Alzheimer's. Rivastigmine (Exelon®): Mild to moderate disease. Galantamine (Razadyne): Mild to moderate disease. | Nausea, vomiting, loss of appetite, and frequent bowel movements. |
| | Tacrine (Cognex®): Mild to moderate disease. | Nausea, vomiting, and possible damage to the liver. |
| **Meman-tine** (Targets glutamate, involved in learning and memory) | Namenda®: Moderate to severe | Headache, confusion, dizziness, and constipation. |

**Assessments**

MMSE and Mini-Cog:
Patients with evidence of dementia or short-term memory loss, often associated with Alzheimer's disease, should have cognition assessed. The Mini-mental state exam (MMSE) or the Mini-cog test is commonly used. Both require the patient to carry out specified tasks.

MMSE:
- Remembering and later repeating the names of 3 common objects.
- Counting backward from 100 by 7s or spelling "world" backward.
- Naming items as the examiner points to them.
- Providing the location of the examiner's office, including city, state, and street address.
- Repeating common phrases.
- Copying a picture of interlocking shapes.
- Following simple 3-part instructions, such a picking up a piece of paper, folding it in half, and placing it on the floor.

Mini-cog:
- Remembering and later repeating the names of 3 common objects.
- Drawing the face of a clock with all 12 numbers and the hands indicating the time specified by the examiner.

Digit Repetition Test:
The Digit Repetition Test is used to assess attention. The patient is told to listen to numbers and then repeat them. The nurse starts with 2 random single-digit numbers. If the patient gets this sequence correct, the nurse then states 3 numbers and continues to add 1 number each time until the patient is unable to repeat the numbers correctly. People with normal intelligence (without mental disability or expressive aphasia) can usually repeat 5 to 7 numbers, so scores ≤ 5 indicate impaired attention.

*Copyright © Mometrix Media. You have been licensed one copy of this document for personal use only. Any other reproduction or redistribution is strictly prohibited. All rights reserved.*

Time and Change Test:
The Time and Change Test assesses dementia in older adults and is effective in diverse populations. Patients are shown a clock face set at 11:10 and have 1 minute to make 2 attempts at stating the correct time. The patient is then given change (7 dimes, 7 nickels, and 3 quarters) and asked to give the nurse $1.00 from the coins. The patient has 2 minutes and 2 tries to make the correct change. Failing either or both tests is indicative of dementia.

## Geriatric Depression Scale

The Geriatric Depression Scale is a self-assessment tool to identify older adults with depression. The test can be used with those with normal cognition and those with mild to moderate impairment. The test poses 15 questions to which a patient answers "yes" or "no." A score of >5 "yes" answers is indicative of depression:

1. Are you basically satisfied with your life?
2. Have you dropped many of your activities and interests?
3. Do you feel your life is empty?
4. Do you often get bored?
5. Are you in good spirits most of the time?
6. Are you afraid that something bad is going to happen to you?
7. Do you feel happy most of the time?
8. Do you often feel helpless?
9. Do you prefer to stay at home rather than going out and doing new things?
10. Do you feel you have more problems with memory than most?
11. Do you think it is wonderful to be alive now?
12. Do you feel pretty worthless the way you are now?
13. Do you feel full of energy?
14. Do you feel that your situation is hopeless?
15. Do you think that most people are better off than you are?

## Depression

Depression is increasingly recognized as a risk factor not only for adults but for children as well. Depression affects about 19% of adults >55 years of age and 37% of older adults with co-morbid conditions, putting older adults (who have the highest rates of suicide) at risk. Depression is associated with conditions that decrease quality of life, such as heart disease, neuromuscular diseases, arthritis, cancer, diabetes, Huntington's disease, and stroke. Some drugs may also precipitate depression: diuretics, drugs used to treat Parkinson's disease, estrogen, corticosteroids, cimetidine, hydralazine, propranolol, digitalis, and indomethacin. Patients with clinical depression experience changes in mood, sadness, loss of interest in usual activities, increased fatigue, change in appetite, fluctuation in weight, anxiety, and sleep disturbance. Adults often have insomnia or sleep excessively; they have trouble concentrating and have feelings of hopelessness. They may become easily angered. Both children and adults may have suicidal thoughts. Depression often goes undiagnosed, so screening for at risk individuals should be done routinely. Usually changes in behavior do become apparent to family members, but these changes may mistakenly be considered symptoms of other medical conditions. *Treatment* includes tricyclic antidepressants (TCAs) and selective serotonin reuptake inhibitors (SSRIs).

## Bipolar disorder

Bipolar disorder causes severe mood swings between hyperactive states and depression, accompanied by impaired judgment because of distorted thoughts. The hypomanic stage may allow for creativity and good functioning in some people, but it can develop into more severe mania, which may be associated with psychosis and hallucinations. There is a subsequent swing into a period of profound depression. Symptoms may be precipitated by environmental triggers, such as medications, stress, substance abuse, sleep disorders, and change of season. Those with late onset (>50 years of age) tend to have less severe symptoms than those with early onset. Bipolar disorder is associated with high rates of suicide, so early diagnosis and treatment is critical. *Intervention* includes both medication (usually given continually) to prevent cycling

*Copyright © Mometrix Media. You have been licensed one copy of this document for personal use only. Any other reproduction or redistribution is strictly prohibited. All rights reserved.*

and control depression and psychotherapy, such as cognitive therapy, which helps patients control disordered thought patterns and behavior. Medications include anticonvulsants, mood stabilizers, atypical antipsychotics, and anti-anxiety medications. Antidepressants are usually contraindicated. Family and group therapy is often useful.

## Borderline personality disorder

Borderline personality disorder (BPD) affects about 2% of adults, mostly young women, but symptoms may begin to develop slowly from about 9 years of age and on into the teen years, resulting in unstable moods and disordered thinking in relation to self-image and behavior. Depression, mood disorders, self-injury, including self-mutilation, and suicide attempts are common, as are drinking and drug use. Patients may perceive themselves as bad and suffer severe separation anxiety and fears. They often engage in impulsive high-risk behaviors, such as promiscuous sex and binge eating. Studies have linked BPD to sexual abuse as children, with 40%-71% of young women diagnosed with BPD victims of sexual abuse during childhood. While definitive diagnosis is usually delayed until young adulthood, because of the associated social and behavioral problems, early recognition of the symptoms and *intervention* with medications and/or behavioral therapy may help the person to effectively cope by developing better behavioral strategies. Medications include mood stabilizers, anti-convulsants, SSRIs, atypical antipsychotics, and opiate receptor antagonists.

## Suicidal patients

Patients may attempt suicide for many reasons, including severe depression, social isolation, situational crisis (job loss, divorce), bereavement, or psychotic disorder (such as schizophrenia). Suspected suicidal patients should be referred for psychiatric evaluation. The initial treatment of a patient who has attempted suicide depends upon the type of suicide attempt. Antidotes for ingestion of common drugs include:

- Opiates: Naloxone (Narcan®).
- Acetaminophen: N-acetylcysteine.

It's important that the family nurse practitioner (FNP) provide support without expressing a negative attitude that may further depress the patient's self-esteem, increasing the risk of further attempts. The patient should be assessed for suicide risk after initial treatment. Those at high risk should be hospitalized. High-risk findings include:

- Violent suicide attempt (knives, gunshots).
- Suicide attempt with low chance of rescue.
- Ongoing psychosis or disordered thinking.
- Ongoing severe depression and feeling of helplessness.
- History of previous suicide attempts.
- Lack of social support system.

## Selective serotonin reuptake inhibitors

Selective serotonin reuptake inhibitors (SSRIs) are antidepressant medications that block the reuptake of serotonin (a neurotransmitter) in the brain, increasing the extracellular level of the neurotransmitter and improving transmission. Drugs include citalopram (Celexa®), escitalopram (Lexapro®), fluoxetine (Prozac®), and paroxetine (Paxil). All SSRIs have similar action but may have different chemical properties that cause various side effects, so some people tolerate one better than another. Side effects include nausea, weight gain, sexual dysfunction, excitation and agitation, insomnia, drowsiness, increased perspiration, headache, and diarrhea. In rare cases, *serotonin syndrome* may occur from high levels of serotonin, from overdose, or from a combination with MAO inhibitors, so SSRIs must not be taken within 2 weeks of each other. Symptoms of serotonin syndrome include severe anxiety and agitation, hallucinations, confusion, blood pressure swings, fever, tachycardia, seizures, and coma. SSRIs are not addictive but abrupt cessation may trigger *discontinuation syndrome* (flu-like symptoms).

*Copyright © Mometrix Media. You have been licensed one copy of this document for personal use only. Any other reproduction or redistribution is strictly prohibited. All rights reserved.*

## Tricyclic antidepressants

Tricyclic antidepressants (named for the 3-ring chemical structure of the first of this group) inhibit the uptake of neurotransmitters, primarily norepinephrine and serotonin, and serve as antagonists to dopamine and histamine. Tricyclic antidepressants usually target 2 or 3 of these neurotransmitters while newer antidepressants, such as SSRIs, target only 1. Tricyclic antidepressants are used to treat depression, ADHD, nocturnal enuresis, and pain (migraine). They are sometimes referred to as cyclic antidepressants because newer drugs have a 4-ring structure. Tricyclic antidepressants are lipophilic and highly protein-bound, so they are absorbed rapidly. Drugs include amitriptyline (Elavil®), imipramine (Tofranil®), and nortriptyline (Aventyl®, Pamelor®). They have long half-lives, which increases toxic effects with overdose and anticholinergic (primarily muscarinic) effects. Because of this, cyclic antidepressants tend to have more side effects than newer antidepressants: dry mouth, blurring vision, cardiac abnormalities, constipation, urinary retention, and hyperthermia. Alterations in memory and cognition, drowsiness, anxiety, muscle twitches, gynecomastia, and breast enlargement may occur. Tricyclic antidepressants are contraindicated with MAO inhibitors and cimetidine.

Overdose:
Tricyclic antidepressants (TCA), such as Elavil® and Tofranil®, cause the most prescription-related deaths. They are prescribed for depression and other psychiatric and medical conditions. Toxicity may result from intentional overdose, excessive therapeutic dose, poly-drug combinations, serotonin syndrome (↑ serotonin in the CNS) and other medical conditions. Symptoms of toxicity vary widely and can include:
- Alterations of consciousness, slurred speech, seizures, coma.
- Dilated or constricted pupils, blurred vision.
- Pulmonary edema.
- Ataxia, tremor, myoclonus, hyperreflexia.

- Tachycardia, hypertension or hypotension, heart block, depressed cardiac contractility.
- ECG: sinus tachycardia with right axis deviation (terminal 40 ms) prolonged PR, QRS, and QT (develop in ≤6 hours).
- Urinary retention and overflow incontinence.

*Diagnosis* includes positive serum TCA and clinical findings, urine drug screening, ECG, serum electrolyte, creatinine, glucose levels, and ABGs. *Treatment* may include IV access, cardiac monitoring, urinary catheter (if necessary), gastric decontamination with gastric lavage (≤1 hour) and charcoal, sodium bicarbonate (to treat dysrhythmias and hypotension), IV dextrose, thiamine, naloxone, barbiturates (to treat seizures), isotonic crystalloid fluids, and/or vasopressors, such as norepinephrine (to treat hypotension).

## Lithium

Lithium carbonate (Eskalith®, Lithobid®) is used to control the manic episodes associated with bipolar disorder. It may also be used in conjunction with antidepressants to treat depression. Lithium has properties similar to sodium and potassium in that it interferes with the action of sodium in neuromuscular cells, reducing agitation. It also interferes with the production and action of neurotransmitters and affects levels of tryptophan and serotonin in the central nervous system. It can also cause an increase in leukocyte production. Lithium crosses the placenta, so it should not be taken during pregnancy or while nursing. Overdosing can cause severe side effects, so blood levels must be routinely monitored. Side effects include hand tremors, twitching, nausea, diarrhea, seizures, confusion, and increase in urinary output. About 1 patient in 25 develops goiter from lithium-induced hypothyroidism. NSAIDs, SSRIs, phenothiazines, and diuretics may cause dangerous drug interactions if taken with lithium.

*Copyright © Mometrix Media. You have been licensed one copy of this document for personal use only.*
*Any other reproduction or redistribution is strictly prohibited. All rights reserved.*

## Rohypnol ingestion

Rohypnol ® (flunitrazepam) is a type of benzodiazepine, commonly referred to as the "date rape drug" or "roofie" because it causes anterograde amnesia. Rohypnol® is popular with teens and young adults and is often taken with alcohol, which potentiates its effects. Rohypnol® is a CNS depressant that causes muscle relaxation, slurs speech and reduces inhibitions. The effects occur within 20-30 minutes of ingestion but may persist for 8 to 12 hours. Repeated use can result in aggressiveness, and withdrawal may cause hallucinations and seizures. Overdosing causes hypotension, altered mental status, vomiting, hallucinations, dyspnea, and coma. *Diagnosis* is by history and clinical examination.

*Treatment* includes

- Assessment for rape (using rape kit, if indicated) with tests for sexually transmitted diseases (STD).
- Gastric emptying (<1 hour).
- Charcoal.
- Monitoring for CNS/respiratory depression.
- Supportive care.
- Flumazenil (antagonist) 0.2 mg each minute to total 3 mg may be used in some cases, but this is not routinely advised because of complications related to benzodiazepine dependency or co-ingestion of cyclic antidepressants.
- Counseling referral for rape.

## Benzodiazepine toxicity

Benzodiazepine toxicity may result from accidental or intentional overdose with such drugs as Xanax®, Librium®, Valium®, Ativan®, Serax®, Versed®, and Restoril®. An outcome of mortality is usually the result of co-ingestion of other drugs. Similarly, coma and severe central nervous depression is usually caused by co-ingestions. *Symptoms* are often non-specific neurological changes: lethargy, dizziness, alterations in consciousness, and ataxia. Respiratory depression and hypotension are rare complications. *Diagnosis* is based on history and clinical exam, as benzodiazepine level does not correlate well with toxicity. *Treatment* includes:

- Gastric emptying (<1 hour).
- Charcoal.
- Concentrated dextrose, thiamine, and naloxone if co-ingestions suspected, especially with altered mental status.
- Monitoring for CNS/respiratory depression.
- Supportive care.
- Flumazenil (antagonist) 0.2 mg each minute. A total of 3 mg may be given in some cases, but it is not routinely advised because of complications related to benzodiazepine dependency or co-ingestion of cyclic antidepressants. Flumazenil is contraindicated in the presence of increased intracranial pressure.

## Substance abuse

Substance abuse in the elderly is often overlooked, but about 10%-15% of older adults abuse alcohol, and many abuse other drugs. Substance abuse is often linked to underlying psychiatric disorders. The most commonly abused drugs include:

- ***Prescription drugs:*** Narcotics and benzodiazepine. Additionally, overuse of prescription drugs is common, especially psychotropics. Benzodiazepine abuse may result in increased falls and auto accidents. The effects are potentiated if taken with alcohol or narcotics. Patients may go through withdrawal and delirium if the medication, especially Xanax, is stopped abruptly.
- ***Non-prescription drugs:*** OTC sleep preparations and alcohol. Alcohol may cause depression-like symptoms, chronic disorders (cirrhosis, cardiomyopathy, and neuropathy), and alcohol brain syndrome. Alcohol use can lead to suicide. Alcohol withdrawal may cause delirium tremens and seizures.
- ***Illicit drugs:*** Marijuana. (Older adults are less likely to use heroin or cocaine).

Substance abuse of prescription drugs is often related to inappropriate or excessive

*Copyright © Mometrix Media. You have been licensed one copy of this document for personal use only. Any other reproduction or redistribution is strictly prohibited. All rights reserved.*

prescriptions. Drug abusers often seek out prescriptions from multiple doctors and may present with dozens of prescribed medications.

Indicators:
Many people with substance abuse (alcohol or drugs) are reluctant to disclose this information, but there are a number of indicators that are suggestive of substance abuse:

| Physical signs | Other signs |
|---|---|
| Needle tracks on arms or legs. Burns on fingers or lips. Pupils abnormally dilated or constricted, eyes watery. Slurring of speech, slow speech. Lack of coordination, instability of gait. Tremors. Sniffing repeatedly, nasal irritation. Persistent cough. Weight loss. Dysrhythmias. Pallor, puffiness of face. | Odor of alcohol/marijuana on clothing or breath. Labile emotions, including mood swings, agitation, and anger. Inappropriate, impulsive, and/or risky behavior. Lying. Missing appointments. Difficulty concentrating/short-term memory loss, disoriented/confused. Blackouts. Insomnia or excessive sleeping. Lack of personal hygiene. |

## CAGE tool

The CAGE tool is used as a quick assessment tool to determine if people are drinking excessively or are problem drinkers. Moderate drinking, (1 drink a day for older adults), unless contraindicated by health concerns, is usually not harmful to people, but drinking more than that can lead to serious psychosocial and physical problems. One drink is defined as 12 ounces of beer/wine cooler, 5 ounces of wine, or 1.5 ounces of liquor.

| C | Cutting down | Do you think about trying to cut down on drinking? |
|---|---|---|
| A | Annoyed at criticism | Are people starting to criticize your drinking? |
| G | Guilty feeling | Do you feel guilty or try to hide your drinking? |
| E | Eye opener | Do you increasingly need a drink earlier in the day? |

"Yes" on one question suggests the possibility of a drinking problem while "yes" on ≥2 questions indicates a drinking problem, and the patient should be provided information about reducing drinking and appropriate referrals made.

## Ethanol

Ethanol is the form of alcohol found in alcoholic beverages, flavorings, and some medications. It is a multisystem toxin and CNS depressant. Teenagers and young adults and those >60 years of age frequently use ethanol as the drug of choice, but binge drinking can lead to serious morbidity or death. Ethanol has direct effects on the central nervous system, myocardium, thyroid, and hepatic tissue. Ethanol is absorbed through the mucosa of the mouth, stomach, and intestines, with concentrations peaking in about 30-60 minutes after ingestion. About 90% of ethanol is metabolized in the liver and the rest excreted through the pulmonary and renal systems. Chronic abuse of ethanol (alcoholism) is also associated with *alcohol withdrawal syndrome (delirium tremens)* when there is an abrupt cessation of alcohol intake, resulting in hallucinations, tachycardia, diaphoresis, and, sometimes, psychotic behavior. Alcohol withdrawal syndrome may be precipitated by trauma or infection and has a high mortality rate, 5%-15% with treatment and 35% without treatment.

Ethanol toxicity:
Ethanol overdose affects the central nervous system as well as other organs in the body. If people are easily aroused, they can usually safely sleep off the effects of ingesting too much alcohol, but if the person is semi-conscious or unconscious, emergency medical treatment should be initiated. Typical *symptoms* include:
- Altered mental status with slurred speech and stupor.

- 103 -

*Copyright © Mometrix Media. You have been licensed one copy of this document for personal use only. Any other reproduction or redistribution is strictly prohibited. All rights reserved.*

- Nausea and vomiting.
- Hypotension.
- Bradycardia with arrhythmias.
- Respiratory depression and hypoxia.
- Cold, clammy skin or flushed skin (from vasodilation).
- Acute pancreatitis with abdominal pain.
- Lack of consciousness.
- Circulatory collapse leading to death.

*Treatment* includes:
- Careful monitoring of arterial blood gases and oxygen saturation.
- Ensure patent airway with intubation and ventilation if necessary.
- Intravenous fluids.
- Dextrose to correct hypoglycemia, if indicated.
- Maintain body temperature (warming blanket).
- Dialysis may be necessary in severe cases.

## Amphetamine and cocaine toxicity

Amphetamine toxicity may be caused by IV injection, inhalation, or insufflation of various substances, which include methamphetamine (MDA or "ecstasy"), methylphenidate (Ritalin®), methylenedioxymethamphetamine (MDMA), and ephedrine and phenylpropanolamine. Cocaine may be ingested orally, IV, or by insufflation, whereas crack cocaine may be smoked. Amphetamines and cocaine are CNS stimulants that can cause multi-system abnormalities. Symptoms may include chest pain, dysrhythmias, myocardial ischemia, MI, seizures, intracranial infarctions, hypertension, dystonia, repetitive movements, unilateral blindness, lethargy, rhabdomyolysis with acute kidney failure, perforated nasal septum (cocaine), and paranoid psychosis (amphetamines). Crack cocaine may cause pulmonary hemorrhage, asthma, pulmonary edema, barotrauma, and pneumothorax. Swallowing packs of cocaine can cause intestinal ischemia, colitis, necrosis, and perforation. Diagnosis includes clinical findings, CBC, chemistry panel, toxicology screening, ECG, and radiograph.

*Treatment* includes:
- Gastric emptying (≤1 hour). Charcoal administration.
- IV access. Supplemental oxygen.
- Sedation for seizures: Lorazepam 2 mg/min IV, diazepam 5 mg IV titrated in repeated doses. Agitation: Haloperidol.
- Hypertension: Nitroprusside, phentolamine 2.5-5 mg IV.
- Cocaine quinidine-like effects: Sodium bicarbonate.

*Copyright © Mometrix Media. You have been licensed one copy of this document for personal use only. Any other reproduction or redistribution is strictly prohibited. All rights reserved.*

# Professional Caring and Ethical Practice

## Synergy model

The synergy model of nursing practice, developed by the ACCN for nursing certification, places the needs of the patient as the central focus and defines the relationship between 8 patient characteristics and 8 nurse competencies. These competencies and characteristics are evaluated on a scale (1-5). *Patient characteristics* include resiliency, vulnerability, stability, complexity, resource availability, participation in care, participation in decision-making, and predictability. *Nurse competencies* include clinical judgment, advocacy, caring practices, collaboration, systems thinking, Response to Diversity, clinical inquiry, and facilitation of learning. The *system or healthcare environment* is the third element of the model. It provides support for the needs of the patients and empowers and nurtures the practice of nursing, caring, and ethical practice. All 3 of these systems are essential for synergy. The needs of the patient are the driving force for nurse competencies, and both are dependent on the healthcare system. When the needs, competencies, and system complement each other, synergy is achieved, and outcomes for the nurse, the patient, and the system are optimized.

Three levels of outcomes:
The ACCN synergy model is based on 3 levels of quality outcomes (patient, nurse, and system). Six general *indicators of quality outcomes* include:
- Satisfaction of patient and family.
- Adverse incidents rates.
- Rate of complications.
- Adherence to discharge plans.
- Mortality rate.
- Length of stay in hospital.

These general outcomes are based on outcomes derived from the patient, the nurse, and the system:

- *Patient outcomes* include functional change, behavioral change, trust, ratings, satisfaction, comfort, and quality of life.
- *Nurse outcomes* include physiological changes, presence or absence of complications, extent to which care or treatment objectives were attained.
- *System outcomes* include recidivism, costs, and resource utilization.

Nurse competencies:
Clinical judgment is using clinical reasoning, decision making, and critical thinking to evaluate a situation and apply skills related to education, experience, knowledge, and evidence-based guidelines in providing care. Clinical judgment includes a thorough knowledge of the nursing process and an ability to utilize data and research. Clinical judgment includes the use of intuition, based on experience and a holistic understanding of all issues involved. Levels of clinical judgment include:
- Level 1: This nurse is at a beginner level and follows algorithms and pathways but cannot vary care according to needs, is able to collect only basic data, and defers to others for some decision-making.
- Level 3: This nurse is competent in collecting and assessing data and can anticipate needs and manage patient care but recognizes different problem levels and may ask for guidance.
- Level 5: This nurse is expert and able to process multiple sources of data and make reasoned decisions about patient care based on knowledge and experience and a holistic view of the patient's needs.

## *Advocacy/Moral Agency*

### Advocacy/moral agency

Nurse competencies under the ACCN synergy model include advocacy/moral agency:
- *Advocacy* is working for the best interests of the patient despite personal values in conflict and assisting patients to have access to appropriate resources.

*Copyright © Mometrix Media. You have been licensed one copy of this document for personal use only. Any other reproduction or redistribution is strictly prohibited. All rights reserved.*

- *Agency* is openness and recognition of issues and a willingness to act.
- *Moral agency* is the ability to recognize needs and take action to influence the outcome of a conflict or decision.

The levels of advocacy/moral agency include
- Level 1:  This nurse works on behalf of the patient, assesses personal values, has awareness of patient's rights and ethical conflicts, and advocates for the patient when consistent with the nurse's personal values.
- Level 3: This nurse advocates for the patient/family, incorporates their values into the care plan even when they differ from the nurse's own, and can utilize internal resources (the current setting) to assist the patient/family with complex decisions.
- Level 5:  This nurse advocates for the patient/family despite differences in values and is able to utilize both internal and external resources (the community at large) to help to empower the patient/family to make decisions.

Approaches:
There are a number of different approaches that can help develop nurses' advocacy and moral agency:
- *Role modeling* takes place when one nurse serves as a role model for others, modeling the behavior and responses that advocate for the patient and show caring practices.
- *Modeling and role modeling* is another concept that is particularly useful in the development of ethical practices. In this case, modeling occurs when the nurse, through observation and interviewing, attempts to gain an understanding of the patient/family's perspective, and then role modeling is using that understanding to assist the patient/family by intervening to ensure that their needs are met.
- *Coaching* involves providing staff with tools, ways to respond or procedures to follow, to help them understand the ways in which they can become an advocate.

- *Mentoring* is providing professional guidance; a staff person brings questions or concerns that relate to her long-range goals to a mentor.

Assessing ethical issues:
While the terms *ethics* and *morals* are sometimes used interchangeably, ethics is a study of morals and encompasses concepts of right and wrong. When making ethical assessments, one must consider not only what people should do but also what they actually do, as these two things are sometimes at odds. Ethical issues can be difficult to assess because of personal bias, and that is one of the reasons that sharing concerns with other internal sources and reaching consensus is so valuable. Issues of concern might include options for care, refusal of care, rights to privacy, adequate relief of suffering, and the right to self-determination. Internal sources might include the ethics committee, whose charge it is to make decisions regarding ethical issues. Risk management can provide guidance related to personal and institutional liability. External agencies might include government agencies, such as the public health department.

**Beneficence and nonmaleficence**

Beneficence is an ethical principle that involves performing actions that are for the purpose of benefiting another person. In the care of a patient, any procedure or treatment should be done with the ultimate goal of benefiting the patient, and any actions that are not beneficial should be reconsidered. As a child ages and/or condition changes, procedures need to be continually reevaluated to determine if they are still of benefit.

Nonmaleficence is an ethical principle that means healthcare workers should provide care in a manner that does not cause direct intentional harm to the patient:
- The actual act must be good or morally neutral.
- The intent must be only for a good effect.
- A bad effect cannot serve as the means to get to a good effect.

*Copyright © Mometrix Media. You have been licensed one copy of this document for personal use only. Any other reproduction or redistribution is strictly prohibited. All rights reserved.*

- A good effect must have more benefit than a bad effect has harm.

## Autonomy and justice

Autonomy is the ethical principle that the individual has the right to make decisions about his/her own care. In the case of children or patients with dementia who cannot make autonomous decisions, parents or family members may serve as the legal decision makers. The nurse must keep the patient and/or family fully informed so that they can exercise their autonomy in informed decision-making. Justice is the ethical principle that relates to the distribution of the limited resources of healthcare benefits to members of society. These resources must be distributed fairly. This issue may arise if there is only 1 bed available and there are 2 sick patients. Justice comes into play in deciding which patient should stay and which should be transported or receive other care. The decision should be made according to what is best or most just for the patients and not influenced by personal bias.

## Bioethics

Bioethics is a branch of ethics that involves making sure that the medical treatment given is the most morally correct choice, given the different options that might be available and the differences inherent in the varied levels of treatment. In the acute/critical care unit, if the patients, parents, and the staff are in agreement when it comes to values and decision-making, then no ethical dilemma exists; however, when there is a difference in value beliefs between the patients/parents and the staff, there is a bioethical dilemma that must be resolved. Sometimes, discussion and explanation can resolve differences, but, at times, the institution's ethics committee must be brought in to resolve the conflict. The primary goal of bioethics is to determine the most morally correct action using the set of circumstances given.

## Informed consent

Patients or guardians must provide informed consent for all treatment the patient receives. This includes a thorough explanation of all procedures and treatments and associated risks. Patients/guardians should be apprised of all options and allowed input on the type of treatments. Patients/guardians should be apprised of all reasonable risks and any complications that might be life threatening or increase morbidity. The American Medical Association has established guidelines for informed consent:
- Explanation of diagnosis.
- Nature and reason for treatment or procedure.
- Risks and benefits.
- Alternative options (regardless of cost or insurance coverage).
- Risks and benefits of alternative options.
- Risks and benefits of not having a treatment or procedure.

Providing informed consent is a requirement of all states.

## Patient/family rights

In order for patient/family rights to be incorporated into the plan of care, the care plan needs to be designed as a collaborative effort that encourages participation of patients and family members. There are a number of different programs that can be useful, such as including patients and families on advisory committees. Additionally, assessment tools, such as surveys for patients/families, can be utilized to gain insight into the issues that are important to them. While infants and small children and sometimes the elderly cannot speak for themselves, "patient" is generally understood to include not only the immediate family but also other groups or communities who have an interest in the care of an individual or individuals. Because many hospital stays are now short term, programs that include follow-up interviews and assessments are especially

Copyright © Mometrix Media. You have been licensed one copy of this document for personal use only. Any other reproduction or redistribution is strictly prohibited. All rights reserved.

valuable in determining if the needs of the patient/family were addressed in the care plan.

## Confidentiality

Confidentiality is the obligation that is present in a professional-patient relationship. Nurses are under an obligation to protect the information they possess concerning the patient and family. Care should be taken to safeguard that information and to provide the privacy that the family deserves. This is accomplished through the use of required passwords when family members call for information about the patient and through the limitation of who is allowed to visit. There may be times when confidentiality must be broken to save the life of a patient, but those circumstances are rare. The nurse practitioner must make all efforts to safeguard patient records and identification. Computerized record keeping should be done in such a way that the screen is not visible to others, and paper records must be secured.

## Empowering patients

Empowering patients and families to act as their own advocates requires they have a clear understanding of their rights and responsibilities. These should be given (in print form) and/or presented (audio/video) to patients and families on admission or as soon as possible thereafter:

- **Rights** should include competent, non-discriminatory medical care that respects privacy and allows participation in decisions about care and the right to refuse care. The patient/family should have clear understandable explanations of treatments, options, and conditions, including outcomes. They should be apprised of transfers, changes in care plan, and advance directives. They should have access to medical records information about charges.
- **Responsibilities** should include providing honest and thorough information about health issues and medical history. The patient/family should ask for clarification if they don't understand information that is

provided to them, and they should follow the plan of care that is outlined or they should explain why that is not possible. They should treat staff and other patients with respect.

## Treating terminally ill patients

There are a number of ethical concerns that healthcare providers and families must face when determining the treatments that are necessary and appropriate for a terminally-ill patient. It is the nurse's responsibility to provide support and information to help parents/families make informed decisions:

- **Caring practices: Advantages** - Provide comfort. Ease the dying process. **Disadvantages**- Increase sedation and decrease cognition and interaction with family. Side effects. May hasten death.
- **Active treatments (such as antibiotics, chemotherapy): Advantages** - Prolong life. Relieve symptoms. Reassure family.
- **Disadvantages** - Prolong the dying process. Side effects may be severe (as with chemotherapy).
- **Supplemental nutrition: Advantages** - Relieve family's anxiety that the child is hungry. Prolong life. **Disadvantages** - May cause nausea, vomiting. May increase tumor growth with cancer. May increase discomfort.
- **IV fluids for hydration: Advantages** - Relieve family's anxiety that the child is thirsty. Keep mouth moist. **Disadvantages** - May result in congestive heart failure and pulmonary edema with increased dyspnea. Increased urinary output and incontinence may cause skin breakdown. Prolong dying process.
- **Resuscitation efforts: Advantages** - Allow family to deny death is imminent. **Disadvantages** - Cause unnecessary suffering and prolong dying process

Copyright © Mometrix Media. You have been licensed one copy of this document for personal use only. Any other reproduction or redistribution is strictly prohibited. All rights reserved.

## Caring Practices

### Caring practices

In the ACCN synergy model, caring practices encompass all nursing activities that respond to the individual patient's and family's needs in a caring, compassionate, and therapeutic environment to promote patient comfort and prevent unnecessary suffering. Caring practices recognize inner strength and its relation to healing and seek to enhance the dignity of the individual through vigilance, nurturance, and skilled technical and basic nursing practices. Levels of caring practices include:

- Level 1: This nurse provides a safe environment and cares for the present basic needs of the patient without focus on future needs and considers death a potential outcome.
- Level 3: This nurse provides compassionate care, responding to changes in the patient and extending acts of kindness while accepting death as a possible outcome and providing measures to ensure good end-of-life care and a peaceful death.
- Level 5: This nurse is fully engaged in patient care and understands and interprets patient/family dynamics and needs, ensuring comfort, dignity, and safety while respecting the individual and family.

### Standards of advance practice

The progressive care nurse is guided by the standards of advance practice, which provides the framework for practice and describes the nurse's responsibilities, related to the values and priorities of the profession:

- **Care process:** In assessing, diagnosing, developing, and implementing a plan of care, as well as evaluating the patient's response, the nurse must use the scientific method and national standards as the basis for care.
- **Establishing priorities:** Providing education and encouraging the patient/family to take an active role in self care is of primary concern. The nurse must

ensure that the patient can make informed decisions. The nurse must assist the patient through all aspects of health care to ensure patient safety and optimal care.

- **Collaboration:** The nurse is a member of the interdisciplinary health team and consults with others when appropriate and refers the patient to specialists as needed. When collaboration is mandated by law, the nurse complies with all requirements.
- **Documentation:** The progressive care nurse keeps accurate, legal, legible records and maintains patient confidentiality. The nurse ensures that the patient signs a release before providing medical records to other parties.
- **Patient advocacy:** The nurse advocates for the individual patient in the process of care but also advocates for patients at the state and national level in order to facilitate patient access to care and improve the quality of care.
- **Continuous quality improvement:** The nurse recognizes the need for constant learning, evaluation, and reevaluation. The nurse participates in quality review and continuing education, thereby maintaining certification at the highest standard of care.
- **Research and education:** The nurse initiates, participates in, and utilizes the results of research in clinical practice.

### Problem solving

Problem solving to anticipate or prevent recurrences of patient/family dissatisfaction involves forming a hypothesis, testing, and assessing data to determine if the hypothesis holds true. If a problem has arisen, taking steps to resolve the immediate problem is only the first step if recurrence is to be avoided:

- **Define the issue:** Talk with the patient or family and staff to determine if the problem related to a failure of communication or other issues, such as differences in culture or religion.
- **Collect data:** This may mean interviewing additional staff or reviewing documentation, gaining a variety of perspectives.

*Copyright © Mometrix Media. You have been licensed one copy of this document for personal use only. Any other reproduction or redistribution is strictly prohibited. All rights reserved.*

- **Identify important concepts:** Determine if there are issues related to values or beliefs.
- **Consider reasons for actions:** Distinguish between motivation and intention on the part of all parties to determine the reason for the problem.
- **Make a decision:** A decision on how to prevent a recurrence of a problem should be based on advocacy and moral agency, reaching the best solution possible for the patient and family.

## Patients' rights

Patient's (family's) rights in relation to what they should expect from a healthcare organization are outlined in the standards of both the Joint Commission and the National Committee for Quality Assurance. Rights include:

- Respect for patient, including personal dignity and psychosocial, spiritual, and cultural considerations.
- Response to needs related to access and pain control.
- Ability to make decisions about care, including informed consent, advance directives, and end of life care.
- Procedure for registering complaints or grievances.
- Protection of confidentiality and privacy.
- Freedom from abuse or neglect.
- Protection during research and information related to the ethical issues of the research.
- Appraisal of outcomes, including unexpected outcomes.
- Information about organizations, services, and practitioners.
- Appeal procedures for decisions regarding benefits and quality of care.
- Organizational code of ethical behavior.
- Procedures for donating and procuring organs/tissue.

## Facilitating safe passage

Facilitating safe passage is the part of caring practice that ensures patient safety, in a broad sense, from a variety of perspectives:

- Giving appropriate medications and treatment without errors that endanger the child's/adult's health is essential.
- Providing information to the patient/family about treatments, changes, conditions, and other aspects related to care helps them cope with situations as they arise.
- Preventing infection is central to patient safety and includes staff using proper infection control methods, such as hand washing.
- Knowing the person being cared for requires the nurse to take the time and effort to understand the needs and wishes of the patient/family.
- Assisting with transitions involves not only helping the patient/family cope with moving from one form of treatment, or one unit to another but also with the transitions in health, such as from illness to health or from illness to death.

## Advance directives

In accordance with Federal and state laws, individuals have the right to self-determination in health care, including decisions about end of life care through advance directives such as living wills and the right to assign a surrogate person to make decisions through a durable power of attorney. Patients should routinely be questioned about an advanced directive because they may present at a healthcare facility without the document. Patients who have indicated they desire a do-not-resuscitate (DNR) order should not receive resuscitative treatments for terminal illness or conditions in which meaningful recovery cannot occur. Patients and families of those with terminal illnesses should be questioned as to whether the patients are hospice patients. For those with DNR requests or those withdrawing life support, staff should provide the patient palliative rather than curative measures, such as pain control and/or oxygen, and emotional support to the patient and family. Religious traditions and beliefs about death should be treated with respect.

*Copyright © Mometrix Media. You have been licensed one copy of this document for personal use only. Any other reproduction or redistribution is strictly prohibited. All rights reserved.*

**Pain management**

Promoting a caring and supportive environment means ensuring that the patient is comfortable. According to Joint Commission guidelines and Federal law, all patients have the right to pain management, and this applies to infants and children. It's not enough to recognize this; procedures must be in place to ensure that all staff is committed to reducing pain and that patients/families are apprised of the right and the benefits of pain management. There are steps that an institution can take in this process:

- Create an interdisciplinary team to research, provide guidelines, and communicate goals.
- Assess pain management procedures already in place to determine effectiveness or need for change.
- Establish minimum standards to be followed that carry legal consequences.
- Clarify responsibility for pain control and imbed this in the standards of practice.
- Provide information about pain control to all levels of care providers.
- Educate patients to understand they are entitled to rapid response.
- Educate staff to institutionalize pain management.

Pain scale:
Pain is subjective and may be influenced by the individual's pain threshold (the smallest stimulus that produces the sensation of pain) and pain tolerance (the maximum degree of pain that a person can tolerate). Currently, the most common pain assessment tool for pre-teens/adolescents is the 1-10 scale:

- 0 = no pain.
- 1-2 = mild pain.
- 3-5 = moderate pain.
- 6-7 = severe pain.
- 8-9 = very severe pain.
- 10 = excruciating pain.

However, there is more to pain assessment than a number on a scale. Assessment includes information about onset, duration, and intensity. Identifying what triggers pain and what relieves it can be very useful when developing a plan for pain management. Patients may show very different behaviors when they are in pain: Some may cry and moan with minor pain, and others may exhibit little difference in behavior when truly suffering. Thus, judging pain by behavior can lead to the wrong conclusion.

Pain Assessment in Advanced Dementia:
Patients with cognitive impairment or inability to verbalize pain may not be able to indicate the degree of pain, even by using a face scale with pictures of smiling to crying faces. The Pain Assessment in Advanced Dementia (PAINAD) scale may be helpful, especially for those with Alzheimer's disease. Careful observation of non-verbal behavior can indicate that the patient is in pain:

- **Respirations**: Patients often have more rapid and labored breathing as pain increases with short periods of hyperventilation or Cheyne-Stokes respirations.
- **Vocalization**: Patients may remain negative in speech or speak quietly and reluctantly. They may moan or groan. As pain increases, they may call out, moan or groan loudly, or cry.
- **Facial expression:** Patients may appear sad or frightened, may frown or grimace, especially on activities that increase pain.
- **Body language:** Patients may be tense, fidget, and pace, and as pain increases, they may become rigid, clench fists, or lie in a fetal position. They may become increasingly combative.
- **Consolability**: Patients are less distractible or consolable with increased pain.

**Supporting families of dying patients**

Often families of dying patients do not receive adequate support from the nursing staff, which feels unprepared for dealing with families' grief and unsure of how to provide comfort, although the families may be in desperate need of this support:

*Copyright © Mometrix Media. You have been licensed one copy of this document for personal use only. Any other reproduction or redistribution is strictly prohibited. All rights reserved.*

| Before death | Stay with the family and sit quietly, allowing them to talk, cry, or interact, if they desire. Avoid platitudes, "His suffering will be over soon." Avoid judgmental reactions to what family members say or do and realize that anger, fear, guilt, and irrational behavior are normal responses to acute grief and stress. Show caring by touching the patient and encouraging family to do the same. Note: Touching hands, arms, or shoulders of family members can provide comfort, but follow the clues of the family. Provide referrals to support groups if available. |
|---|---|

The family requires much support when the patient dies:

| Time of death | Reassure the family that all measures have been taken to ensure the patient's comfort. Express personal feeling of loss, "She was such a sweet woman, and I'll miss her" and allow family to express feelings and memories. Provide information about what is happening during the dying process, explaining death rales, Cheyne-Stokes respirations, etc. Alert family members to imminent death if they are not present. Assist to contact clergy/spiritual advisors. Respect feelings and needs of spouse, parents, siblings, and other family members. |
|---|---|
| After death | Encourage spouse/parents/family members to stay with the patient as long as they wish to say goodbye. Use the patient's name when talking to the family. |

| | Assist family to make arrangements, such as contacting a funeral home. If an autopsy is required, discuss it with the family and explain when it will take place. If organ donation is to occur, assist the family to make arrangements. Encourage family members to grieve and express emotions. Send card or condolence note. |
|---|---|

**Kübler-Ross's 5 stages of grief**

Grief is a normal response to the death or severe illness/abnormality of a patient. How a person deals with grief is very personal, and each will grieve differently. Elisabeth Kübler-Ross identified 5 **stages of grief** in *On Death and Dying* (1969), which can apply to both patients and family members. A person may not go through each stage but usually goes through 2 of the 5 stages:

- **Denial**: Patients/families may be resistive to information and unable to accept that a person is dying/impaired. They may act stunned, immobile, or detached and may be unable to respond appropriately or remember what's said, often repeatedly asking the same questions.
- **Anger**: As reality becomes clear, patient/families may react with pronounced anger, directed inward or outward. Women, especially, may blame themselves, and self-anger may lead to severe depression and guilt, assuming they are to blame because of some personal action. Outward anger, more common in men, may be expressed as overt hostility.

The last 3 stages of Kübler-Ross's 5 stages of grief (after denial and anger) include:

- **Bargaining**: This involves if-then thinking (often directed at a deity): "If I go to church every day, then God will prevent this." Patient/family may change doctors, trying to change the outcome.

*Copyright © Mometrix Media. You have been licensed one copy of this document for personal use only. Any other reproduction or redistribution is strictly prohibited. All rights reserved.*

- *Depression*: As the patient and family begin to accept the loss, they may become depressed, feeling no one understands and overwhelmed with sadness. They may be tearful or crying and may withdraw or ask to be left alone.
- *Acceptance*: This final stage represents a form of resolution and often occurs outside of the medical environment. After a time, patients are able to accept the prospect of their own death/dying. Months after a death, families are able to resume their normal activities and lose the constant preoccupation with their loved one. They are able to think of the person without severe pain.

## Medication errors

About 7000 deaths yearly in the United States are attributed to medication errors. Studies indicate that errors typically occur in 1 of 5 doses of medication given to patients in hospitals. A caring environment is one in which patient safety is ensured with proper handling and administering of medications, as shown:

- Avoiding error-prone abbreviations or symbols. The Joint Commission has established a list of abbreviations to avoid, but mistakes are frequent with other abbreviations as well. In many cases, abbreviations and symbols should be avoided altogether or restricted to a limited approved list.
- Preventing errors from illegible handwriting. Handwritten orders should be block-printed to reduce chance of error.
- Instituting bar coding and scanners that allow the patient's wristband and medications to be scanned for verification.
- Providing lists of similarly-named medications to the staff so that they are well informed.
- Establishing an institutional policy for administering of medications that includes protocols for drug verification, dosage, and patient, as well as educating the patient about the medications.

## Therapeutic communication

Therapeutic communication begins with respect for the patient/family and the assumption that all communication, verbal and non-verbal, has meaning. Listening must be done empathetically. Techniques that facilitate communication include:

| | |
|---|---|
| *Introduction* | Make a personal introduction and use the patient's name: "Mrs. Brown, I am Susan Williams, your nurse." |
| *Encouragement* | Use an open-ended opening statement: "Is there anything you'd like to discuss?" Acknowledge comments: "Yes," and "I understand." Allow silence and observe non-verbal behavior rather than trying to force the conversation. Ask for clarification if the patient's statements are unclear. Reflect statements back (use sparingly): Patient: "I hate this hospital." Nurse: "You hate this hospital?" |
| *Empathy* | Make observations: "You are shaking," and "You seem worried." Recognize feelings: Patient: "I want to go home." Nurse: "It must be hard to be away from your home and family." Provide information as honestly and completely as possible about condition, treatment, and procedures and respond to patient's questions and concerns. |
| *Exploration* | Verbally express implied messages: Patient: "This treatment is too much trouble." Nurse: "You think the treatment isn't helping you?" Explore a topic but allow the patient to terminate the discussion without further probing: "I'd |

*Copyright © Mometrix Media. You have been licensed one copy of this document for personal use only. Any other reproduction or redistribution is strictly prohibited. All rights reserved.*

| | |
|---|---|
| | like to hear how you feel about that. |
| *Orientation* | Indicate reality: Patient: "Someone is screaming." Nurse: "That sound was an ambulance siren." Comment on distortions without directly agreeing or disagreeing: Patient: "That nurse promised I didn't have to walk again." Nurse: "Really? That's surprising because the doctor ordered physical therapy twice a day." |
| *Collaboration* | Work together to achieve better results: "Maybe if we talk about this, we can figure out a way to make the treatment easier for you." |
| *Validation* | Seek validation: "Do you feel better now?" or "Did the medication help you breathe better." |

Avoiding non-therapeutic communication: While using therapeutic communication is important, it is equally important to avoid interjecting non-therapeutic communication, which can block effective communication. *Avoid the following:*

- Meaningless clichés: "Don't worry. Everything will be fine." "Isn't it a nice day?"
- Providing advice: "You should…" or "The best thing to do is…." It's better when patients ask for advice to provide facts and encourage the patient to reach a decision.
- Inappropriate approval that prevents the patient from expressing true feeling or concerns:
  - o Patient: "I shouldn't cry about this."
  - o Nurse: "That's right! You're an adult!"
- Asking for explanations of behavior that is not directly related to patient care and that requires analysis and explanation of feelings: "Why are you upset?"

- Agreeing with, rather than accepting and responding to patient's statements, can make it difficult for the patient to change his/her statement or opinion later: "I agree with you," or "You are right."
- Negative judgments: "You should stop arguing with the nurses."
- Devaluing patient's feelings: "Everyone gets upset at times."
- Disagreeing directly: "That can't be true," or "I think you are wrong."
- Defending against criticism: "The doctor is not being rude; he's just very busy today."
- Subject change to avoid dealing with uncomfortable topics;
  - o Patient: " I'm never going to get well."
  - o Nurse: "Your family will be here in just a few minutes."
- Inappropriate literal responses, even as a joke, especially if the patient is at all confused or having difficulty expressing ideas:
  - o Patient: "There are bugs crawling under my skin."
  - o Nurse: "I'll get some bug spray,"
- Challenge to establish reality often just increases confusion and frustration:
  - o "If you were dying, you wouldn't be able to yell and kick!"

## *Collaboration*

### Collaboration

In the ACCN synergy model, Collaboration is a team approach of working with a variety of others (physicians, nurses, dieticians, therapist, families, social workers, community leaders and members, clergy, intra- and inter-disciplinary teams) in a cooperative manner, using good therapeutic communication skills, to ensure that each person is contributing optimally toward reaching the patient's goals and positive outcomes. Collaboration requires mutual respect, professional maturity, common purpose, and a positive sense of self. Levels of collaboration include:

*Copyright © Mometrix Media. You have been licensed one copy of this document for personal use only. Any other reproduction or redistribution is strictly prohibited. All rights reserved.*

- Level 1: This nurse participates in collaborative activities, learns from others, including mentors, and respects the input of others.
- Level 3: This nurse not only participates in collaborative activities but also initiates them and actively seeks learning opportunities.
- Level 5: This nurse takes a leadership role in collaborative activities by mentoring and teaching others while still seeking learning opportunities and actively seeking additional resources, as needed.

Skills needed:

Nurses must learn the set of skills needed for collaboration in order to move nursing forward. Nurses must take an active role in gathering data for evidence-based practice to support nursing's role in health care, and they must share this information with other nurses and health professionals in order to plan staffing levels and to provide optimal care to patients. Increased and adequate staffing has consistently been shown to reduce adverse outcomes, but there is a well-documented shortage of nurses in the United States, and more than half of current RNs work outside the hospital. Increased patient loads not only increase adverse outcomes but also increase job dissatisfaction and burnout. In order to manage the challenges facing nursing, nurses must develop skills needed for collaboration:

- Be willing to compromise.
- Communicate clearly. Specific challenges and problems.
- Focus on the task.
- Work with teams.

**Delegation of tasks**

Unlicensed assistive personnel:

The scope of nursing practice includes delegation of tasks to unlicensed assistive personnel, provided those individuals have adequate training and knowledge to carry out the tasks. Delegation should be used to manage the workload and to provide adequate and safe care. The nurse who delegates remains accountable for patient outcomes and for supervision of the person to whom the task was delegated, so the nurse must consider the following:

- Whether the knowledge, skills, and training of the unlicensed assistive personnel provides the ability to perform the delegated task.
- Whether the patient's condition and needs have been properly evaluated and assessed.
- Whether the nurse is able to provide ongoing supervision.

Delegation should be done in a manner that reduces liability by providing adequate communication. This includes specific directions about the task, including what needs to be done, when, and for how long. Expectations related to consultation, reporting, and completion of tasks should be clearly defined. The nurse should be available to assist, if necessary.

Teams:

One major responsibility of leadership and management in performance improvement teams is using delegation effectively. The purpose of having a team is having the work shared, and leaders can cripple themselves by taking on too much of the workload. Additionally, failure to delegate shows an inherent distrust in team members. Delegation includes:

- Assessing the skills and available time of the team members, determining if a task is suitable for an individual.
- Assigning tasks, with clear instructions that include explanation of objectives and expectations, including a timeline.
- Ensuring that the tasks are completed properly and on time by monitoring progress but not micromanaging.
- Reviewing the final results and recording the outcomes.

Because the leader is ultimately responsible for the delegated work, mentoring, monitoring, and providing feedback and intervention, as necessary, during this process are necessary components of good leadership. While delegated

Copyright © Mometrix Media. You have been licensed one copy of this document for personal use only. Any other reproduction or redistribution is strictly prohibited. All rights reserved.

tasks may not always be completed successfully, they represent an opportunity for learning.

## Vision of care

Facilitating the creation of a common vision for care within the healthcare system begins with the organization/facility working collaboratively to create teams and an organization focused on serving the patient/family. A common vision should be the ideal in any organization, but achieving such a goal requires a true collaborative effort:

- Inclusion of all levels of staff across the organization/facility, both those in nursing and non-nursing positions.
- Consensus building through discussions, in-service, and team meetings to bring about convergence of diverse viewpoints.
- Facilitation that values creativity and provides encouragement during the process.
- Preparation of a vision statement incorporating the common vision that is accessible to all staff.

Recognition that a common vision is an organic concept that may evolve over time and should be reevaluated regularly and changed, as needed, to reflect the needs of the organization, patients, families, and staff.

## Teambuilding

Leading, facilitating, and participating in performance improvement teams requires a thorough understanding of the dynamics of team building:

- *Initial interactions:* This is when members begin to define their roles and develop relationships, determining if they are comfortable in the group.
- *Power issues:* The members observe the leader and determine who controls the meeting and how control is exercised; members are beginning to form alliances.
- *Organizing:* Methods for accomplishing work are clarified and team members begin to work together, gaining respect for each other's contributions and working toward a common goal.
- *Team identification:* Interactions often become less formal as members develop rapport and are more willing to help and support each other to achieve goals.
- *Excellence:* This develops through a combination of good leadership, committed team members, clear goals, high standards, a spirit of collaboration, a shared commitment to the process, and external recognition.

Techniques:
Leading and facilitating improvement teams requires utilizing good techniques for meetings. Considerations include:

- *Scheduling:* Both the time and the place must be convenient and conducive to working together, so the leader must review the work schedules of those involved, finding the most convenient time. Venues or meeting rooms should allow for sitting in a circle or around a table to facilitate equal exchange of ideas. Any necessary technology, such as computers, overhead projectors, or other equipment should be available.
- *Preparation:* The leader should prepare a detailed agenda that includes a list of items for discussion.
- *Conduction:* Each item of the agenda should be discussed, soliciting input from all group members. Tasks should be assigned to individual members based on their interest and their part in the process of preparing for the next meeting. The leader should summarize input and begin a tentative future agenda.
- *Observation:* The leader should observe the interactions, both verbal and non-verbal communication, and respond to these.

## Leading teams

There are a number of skills that are needed to lead and facilitate coordination of intradisciplinary and interdisciplinary teams:

- Communicating openly is essential with all members encouraged to participate as valued members of a cooperative team.

*Copyright © Mometrix Media. You have been licensed one copy of this document for personal use only.*
*Any other reproduction or redistribution is strictly prohibited. All rights reserved.*

- Avoiding interrupting or interpreting the point another is trying to make allows free flow of ideas.
- Avoiding jumping to conclusions, which can effectively shut off communication.
- Active listening requires paying attentions and asking questions for clarification rather than challenging another's ideas.
- Respecting others' opinions and ideas, even when opposed to one's own, is absolutely essential.
- Reacting and responding to facts rather than feelings allows one to avoid angry confrontations or diffuse anger.
- Clarifying information or opinions stated can help avoid misunderstandings.
- Keeping unsolicited advice out of the conversation shows respect for others and allows them to solicit advice without feeling pressured.

**Leadership styles**

Leadership styles often influence the perception of leadership values and commitment to collaboration. There are a number of different leadership styles:

| | |
|---|---|
| *Charismatic* | Depends upon personal charisma to influence people and may be very persuasive, but this type of leadership may engage "followers" and relating to one group rather than the organization at large, limiting effectiveness. |
| *Bureaucratic* | Follows organization rules exactly and expects everyone else to do so. This is most effective in handling cash flow or managing work in dangerous work environments. This type of leadership may engender respect but may not be conducive to change. |
| *Autocratic* | Makes decisions independently and strictly enforces rules, but team members often feel left out of the process and may not be supportive. This type of leadership is most effective in crisis situations but may have difficulty gaining commitment of staff |
| *Consultative* | Presents a decision and welcomes input and questions, although decisions rarely change. This type of leadership is most effective when gaining the support of staff is critical to the success of the proposed changes. |
| *Participatory* | Presents a potential decision and then makes a final decision based on input from staff or teams. This type of leadership is time-consuming and may result in compromises that are not wholly satisfactory to the management or staff, but this process is motivating to the staff because their expertise is valued. |
| *Democratic* | Presents a problem and asks staff or teams to arrive at a solution although the leader usually makes the final decision. This type of leadership may delay decision-making, but the staff and teams are often more committed to the solutions because of their input. |
| *Laissez-fair (free rein)* | Exerts little direct control but allows employees/teams to make decisions with little interference. This may be effective leadership if the teams are highly skilled and motivated, but, in many cases, this type of leadership is the product of poor management skills, and little is accomplished because of this lack of leadership. |

Copyright © Mometrix Media. You have been licensed one copy of this document for personal use only. Any other reproduction or redistribution is strictly prohibited. All rights reserved.

## Resistance to organizational change

Performance improvement processes cannot occur without organizational change, and resistance to change is common for many people. Therefore, coordinating collaborative processes requires anticipating resistance and taking steps to achieve cooperation. Resistance often relates to concerns about job loss and increased responsibilities, or reflects general denial, lack of understanding, or frustration. Leaders can empower others involved in the process of change by taking these steps:

- Be honest, informative, and tactful, giving people complete information about anticipated changes and how the changes will affect them. Include the positives.
- Be patient and allow people the time they need to contemplate changes and express anger or disagreement.
- Be empathetic and listen carefully to the concerns of others.
- Encourage participation, allowing staff to propose methods of implementing change, so they feel some sense of ownership.
- Establish a climate in which all staff members are encouraged to identify needs for change on an ongoing basis.
- Present further ideas for change to management.

## Conflict resolution

Conflict is an almost inevitable product of teamwork, and the leader must assume responsibility for conflict resolution. While conflicts can be disruptive, they can produce positive outcomes by forcing team members to listen to different perspectives and by opening a dialogue. The team should make a plan for dealing with conflict resolution. The best time for conflict resolution is when differences emerge but before open conflict and hardening of positions occur. The leader must pay close attention to the people and problems involved, listen carefully, and reassure all that their points of view are understood. Steps to conflict resolution include:

- Allow both sides to present their side of the conflict without bias, maintaining a focus on opinions rather than individuals.
- Encourage cooperation through negotiation and compromise.
- Maintain the focus, providing guidance to keep the discussions on track, avoiding spurious arguments.
- Evaluate the need for renegotiation, formal resolution process, or third party.
- Utilize humor and empathy to diffuse escalating tensions.
- Summarize the issues, outlining key arguments.
- Avoid forcing the resolution if possible.

## Collaboration with patient

One of the most important forms of collaboration is that between the nurse and the patient/family, but this type of collaboration is often overlooked. Nurses and others in the healthcare team must always remember that the point of collaborating is to improve patient care, and this means that the patient and patient's family must remain central to all planning. For example, including the family in planning for a patient takes time initially, but sitting down and asking the patient and family, "What do you want?" and using the synergy model to evaluate the patient's (and family's) characteristics can provide valuable information that facilitates planning and, in the long run, saves time and the expenditure of resources. Families, and even young children, often want to participate in care and planning, and they feel validated and more positive toward the medical system when they are included.

Staffing needs:

As nursing resources become more limited, staffing must be done efficiently to best meet the needs of patients. The synergy model can be used in a collaborative effort to identify those patients who are most in need of care. This requires observation and evidence-based research. Often, different units use different criteria to determine staffing needs, but the

Copyright © Mometrix Media. You have been licensed one copy of this document for personal use only. Any other reproduction or redistribution is strictly prohibited. All rights reserved.

synergy model can be used across disciplines and in different types of units. For example, one hospital used the synergy model to determine which patients required a 1:1 patient-staff ratio in the critical care unit. When considering the patient characteristics (resiliency, vulnerability, stability, complexity, resource availability, participation in care, participation in decision-making, and predictability), the staff determined that 4 characteristics (stability, complexity, vulnerability, and resiliency) at Level 1 could be used as the determinant for 1:1 twenty-four-hour care. Those at Levels 2 and 3 required fewer hours of 1:1 care so that the nurse could also care for other patients.

## Communication skills

Collaboration requires a number of communication skills that differ from those involved in communication between nurse and patient. These skills include:

- *Using an assertive approach:* It's important for the nurse to honestly express opinions and to state them clearly and with confidence, but the nurse must do so in a calm, non-threatening manner.
- *Making casual conversation:* It's easier to communicate with people with whom one has a personal connection. Asking open-ended questions, asking about another's work, or commenting on someone's contributions helps to establish a relationship. The times before meetings, during breaks, and after meetings are opportunities for this type of conversation.
- *Being competent in public speaking:* Collaboration requires that a nurse be comfortable speaking and presenting ideas to groups of people and doing so helps that nurse gain credibility. This is a skill that must be practiced.
- *Communicating in writing:* The written word remains a critical component of communication, and the nurse should be able to communicate clearly and grammatically.

## *Systems Thinking*

### Systems thinking

In the ACCN synergy model, systems thinking is having the background knowledge and practical tools to manage both environmental and system resources, within and outside of the healthcare system, to solve problems for the patient/family and meet their needs. Solving problems requires a holistic view of interrelationships and an understanding of how structures, patterns, and events affect outcomes. Levels of systems thinking include:

- Level 1: This nurse views himself/herself as the primary resource to meet the needs of the patient within the confines of the unit and doesn't recognize the need to negotiate.
- Level 3: This nurse looks beyond the unit and personal contributions to care to view the patient's progress through the entire system and sees the need to negotiate with others to provide the best resources available, although the nurse may lack the skills needed to do so.
- Level 5: This nurse is an expert at understanding the organization holistically and uses a number of different strategies to negotiate with others and assist the patient with progress through the system.

### Patient characteristics

The synergy method for patient care recognizes that there are a number of patient characteristics that must be considered if a nurse's competencies are to match those of the patient/family:

- *Resiliency* is the ability to recover from a devastating illness and regain a sense of stability, both physically and emotionally. Things that often support resiliency are faith, continued hope, and a supportive network of friends and family.
- *Vulnerability* refers to factors that put a person at increased risk and interfere with recovery and/or compliance, such as anxiety,

*Copyright © Mometrix Media. You have been licensed one copy of this document for personal use only. Any other reproduction or redistribution is strictly prohibited. All rights reserved.*

fear, lack of support, chronic illness, prejudice, and lack of information.

- **Stability** allows a patient/family to maintain a state of equilibrium (physically and/or emotionally) despite illness and challenges. Important factors include relief from stress, conflicts, and emotional burdens as well as motivation and values.
- **Complexity** occurs when more than one system is involved. These can be internal (cardiac and renal) systems or external (addicted and homeless) systems or a combination of the two (ill with poor family dynamics).

## Barriers to systems thinking

Barriers to system thinking can arise with the individual, the department, or the administrative level:

- **Identification with role rather than purpose**: People see themselves from the perspective of their role in the system, as nurse or physician, and are not able to step outside their preconceived ideas to view situations holistically or to accept the roles of others. They may lack the ability to look at situations as human beings first and professionals second.
- **Feelings of victimization:** People may blame the organization or the leadership for personal shortcomings or feel that there is nothing that they can do to improve or change situations. A feeling of victimization may permeate an institution to the point that meaningful communication cannot take place, and people are not open to change.
- **Relying on past experience:** New directions require new solutions, so being mired in the past or relying solely on past experience can prevent progress.
- **Autocratic views:** Some individuals feel that their perceptions and practices are the only ones that are acceptable and often have a narrow focus so that they cannot view the system as a whole but focus on short-term outcomes. They fail to see that there are many aspects to a problem, affecting many parts of the system.

- **Failure to adapt:** Change is difficult for many individuals and institutions, but the medical world is changing rapidly, and this requires adaptability. Those who fail to adapt may feel threatened by changes and unsure of their ability to relearn new concepts, principles, and procedures.
- **Weak consensus:** Groups that arrive at easy or weak consensus without delving into important issues may delude themselves into believing that they have solved their problems. Rather than moving forward, however, they may have remained fixed, with crucial issues often ignored.

## Delivery of care

The delivery of care is impacted by numerous forces:

- **Social forces** are an increasing demand for access to treatment and medical services, both traditional and complementary. Because society views equitable medical care as a right, the delivery of care must be made available to all.
- **Political forces** are affecting medical care to an increasing degree as the Federal and state governments increasingly become purchasers of medical care. They are also imposing their guidelines and limitations on the medical system.
- **Regulatory forces** may be local, state, or Federal and can have a profound effect on the delivery of care and services, which differ from one state or region to another.
- **Economic forces**, such as managed care or cost-containment committees, try to contain costs to insurers and facilities by controlling access to and the duration of treatment and by limiting products. Economic pressure is working to prevent duplication of services in a geographical area, and providers are creating networks to purchase supplies and equipment directly.

## Systems thinking concepts

The promotion of organizational values and commitment requires that the organization

Copyright © Mometrix Media. You have been licensed one copy of this document for personal use only. Any other reproduction or redistribution is strictly prohibited. All rights reserved.

embody systems thinking and its associated concepts. Systems thinking focuses on how systems interrelate, with each part affecting the entire system: Concepts include:

- **Individual responsibility**: Individuals are encouraged to establish their own goals within the organization and to work toward a purpose.
- **Learning process:** The internalized beliefs of the staff are respected while building upon these beliefs to establish a mindset based on continuous learning and improvement.
- **Vision**: A sharing of organizational vision helps staff to understand the purpose of change and builds commitment.
- **Team process:** Teams are assisted in developing good listening and collaborative skills so that there is an increase in dialogue and an ability to reach consensus.
- **Systems thinking:** Staff members are encouraged to understand the interrelationship of all members of the organization and to appreciate how any change affects the whole.

Steps to systems thinking:
An approach to systems thinking is especially valuable in organizations in which there is lack of consensus, effective change is stalemated, and standards are inconsistent. Systems thinking is a critical thinking approach to problem solving that takes an organization-wide perspective. Steps include:

- **Define the issue:** Describe the problem in detail without judgment or solutions.
- **Describe behavior patterns:** This includes listing factors related to the problem, using graphs to outline possible trends.
- **Establish cause-effect relationships:** This may include using the Five Whys or other root cause analysis or feedback loops.
- **Define patterns of performance/behavior:** Determine how variables affect outcomes and the types of patterns of behavior currently taking place.
- **Find solutions:** Discuss possible solutions and outcomes.

- **Institute performance improvement activities:** Make changes and then monitor for changes in behavior.

## Key quality concepts

There are a number of key concepts related to quality that must be communicated to all members of an organization through in-service workshops, newsletters, fact sheets, and team meetings. Quality care/performance should be:

- **Appropriate** to needs and in keeping with best practices.
- **Accessible** to the individual despite financial, cultural, or other barriers.
- **Competent** with practitioners well-trained and adhering to standards.
- **Coordinated** among all healthcare providers.
- **Effective** in achieving outcomes based on the current state of knowledge.
- **Efficient** in methods of achieving the desired outcomes.
- **Preventive**, allowing for early detection and prevention of problems.
- **Respectful** and caring with consideration of individual needs given primary importance.
- **Safe** so that the organization is free of hazards or dangers that may put patients or others at risk.

## Response to Diversity

### Response to Diversity

In the ACCN synergy model, Response to Diversity is the ability to recognize a wide range of differences (social, cultural, ethnic, racial, economic, language, and religious), to appreciate these differences, and incorporate consideration for them into the plan of care. Diverse groups also include the disabled, gay and lesbians, and marginal groups, such as the homeless. Levels of Response to Diversity include:

- Level 1: This nurse can assess diversity with standardized questionnaires and provide care based on personal belief system and past experience, but doesn't seek assistance in dealing adequately with diversity.

*Copyright © Mometrix Media. You have been licensed one copy of this document for personal use only. Any other reproduction or redistribution is strictly prohibited. All rights reserved.*

- Level 3: This nurse takes a much more active role in asking about issues of diversity and incorporates the patient's needs into the plan of care, teaching the patient about the healthcare system.
- Level 5: This nurse considers issues of diversity in all aspects of care and presents patients with alternatives by responding to, anticipating, and integrating consideration of cultural and other differences.

## Cultural competence

Difference cultures view health and illness from very different perspectives, and patients often come from a mix of many cultures, so the acute care nurse must be not only accepting of cultural differences but sensitive and aware. There are a number of characteristics that are important in order for a nurse to have cultural competence:

- *Appreciating diversity:* This must be grounded in information about other cultures and an understanding of their value system.
- *Assessing own cultural perspectives:* Self-awareness is essential to understanding potential biases.
- *Understanding intercultural dynamics:* This must include understanding ways in which cultures cooperate, differ, communicate, and reach understanding.
- *Recognizing institutional culture:* Each institutional unit (hospital, clinic, office) has an inherent set of values that may be unwritten but is accepted by the staff.
- *Adapting patient service to diversity:* This is the culmination of cultural competence as it is the point of contact between cultures.

## Cultural sensitivities

Jehovah Witnesses:
Jehovah Witnesses have traditionally shunned transfusions and blood products as part of their religious belief. When medical care indicates the need for blood transfusion or blood products and the patient and/or family members are practicing Jehovah Witnesses, this may present a conflict. It's important to approach the patient/family with full information and reasons for the transfusion or blood components without being judgmental, allowing them to express their feelings. In fact, studies show that while adults often refuse transfusions for themselves, they frequently allow their children to receive blood products, so one should never assume that an individual would refuse blood products based on the person's religion alone. In 2004, the *Watchtower,* a Jehovah Witness publication, presented a guide for members. The following guidelines were provided, indicating that Jehovah Witnesses can receive fractionated blood cells, thus allowing hemoglobin-based blood substitutes:

| Basic blood standards for Jehovah Witnesses | |
|---|---|
| **Not acceptable** | Whole blood: red cells, white cells, platelets, plasma |
| **Acceptable** | Fractions from red cells, white cells, platelets, and plasma |

Mexican patients:
Many areas of the country have large populations of Mexican and Mexican-Americans. As always, it's important to recognize that cultural generalizations don't always apply to individuals. Recent immigrants, especially, have cultural needs that the nurse must understand:

- Most Mexicans are Catholic and may like the nurse to make arrangements for a priest to visit.
- Large extended families may come to visit to support the patient and family, so patients should receive clear explanations about how many visitors are allowed, but some flexibility may be required.
- Language barriers may exist because some Mexicans may have limited or no English skills. Translation services should be available around the clock.
- Mexican culture encourages outward expressions of emotions. The family may react strongly to news about a patient's condition, and people who are ill may expect some degree of pampering, so extra attention to the patient/family members may alleviate some of their anxiety.

Copyright © Mometrix Media. You have been licensed one copy of this document for personal use only. Any other reproduction or redistribution is strictly prohibited. All rights reserved.

- Some immigrant Mexicans have very little formal education, so medical information may seem very complex and confusing, and they may not understand the implications or need for follow-up care.
- Mexican culture perceives time with more flexibility than American, so if parents need to be present at a particular time, the nurse should specify the exact time (1:30 PM) and explain the reason rather than saying something more vague, such as "after lunch."
- People may appear to be unassertive or unable to make decisions when they are simply showing respect to the nurse by being deferent.
- In traditional families, the males make decisions, so a woman may wait for the father or other males in the family to make decisions about treatment or care.
- Families may choose to use folk medicines instead of Western medical care or may combine the two.
- Children and young women are often sheltered and are taught to be respectful to adults, so they may not express their needs openly.

## Middle Eastern patients

There are considerable cultural differences among Middle Easterners, but religious beliefs about the segregation of males and females are common. It's important to remember that segregating the female is meant to protect her virtue. Female nurses have low status in many countries because they violate this segregation by touching male bodies, so parents may not trust or show respect for the nurse who is caring for their family member. Additionally, male patients may not want to be cared for by female nurses or doctors, and families may be very upset at a female being cared for by a male nurse or physician. When possible, these cultural traditions should be accommodated:

- In Middle Eastern countries, males make decisions, so issues for discussion or decision should be directed to males, such as the father or spouse, and males may be direct in stating what they want, sometimes appearing demanding.
- If a male nurse must care for a female patient, then the family should be advised that *personal care* (such as bathing) will be done by a female nurse while the medical treatments will be done by the male nurse.
- Families may practice strict dietary restrictions, such as avoiding pork and requiring that animals be killed in a ritual manner, so vegetarian or kosher meals may be required.
- People may have language difficulties and require a translator. Same-sex translators should be used, if at all possible.
- Families may be accompanied by large extended families. Everyone should be kept informed so that they can participate in any discussions that take place before decisions are made.
- Most medical care is provided by female relatives, so educating the family about patient care should be directed to the women in the family (with female translators, if necessary).
- Outward expressions of grief are considered ways of showing respect for the dead.
- Middle Eastern families often offer gifts to caregivers. Small gifts (candy) should be accepted graciously, but for other gifts, the families should be advised graciously that accepting gifts is against hospital policy.
- Middle Easterners often require less personal space and may stand very close.

## Asian patients

There are considerable differences among different Asian populations, so cultural generalizations may not apply to all, but nurses caring for Asian patients should be aware of certain common cultural attitudes and behaviors:

- Nurses and doctors are viewed with respect, so traditional Asian families may expect the nurse to remain authoritative and to give directions that they may not question. The nurse should ensure that information is

*Copyright © Mometrix Media. You have been licensed one copy of this document for personal use only. Any other reproduction or redistribution is strictly prohibited. All rights reserved.*

understood by having the family review the material with her. The nurse should give demonstrations and provide clear explanations, anticipating questions that the family might have but not articulate.

- Disagreeing is considered impolite. "Yes" may only mean that the person is heard, not that they agree with the person. When asked if they understand, they may indicate that they do even when they clearly do not, to avoid offending the nurse.
- Asians may avoid eye contact as an indication of respect. This is especially true of children in relation to adults.
- Patients/families may not show outward expressions of feelings/grief, sometimes appearing passive. They also avoid public displays of affection. This does not mean that their feelings are any less, just that they don't show their feelings.
- Families often hide illness and disabilities from others and may feel ashamed about illness.
- Terminal illness is often hidden from the patient, so families may not want patients to know they are dying or seriously ill.

- Families may use cupping, pinching, or applying pressure to injured areas, and this can leave bruises that may appear as abuse. Thus, when bruises are found, the family should be questioned about the use of alternative therapy before assumptions are made.
- Patients may be treated with traditional herbs.
- Families may need translators because of little or no English skills.
- In traditional Asian families, men are authoritative and make the decisions.

## Clinical Inquiry

### Clinical inquiry

Clinical inquiry is a continual process of questioning and evaluating practice in order to provide innovative and outstanding care through application of the results of research and experience. Clinical inquiry requires a desire to acquire new knowledge, openness to accepting advice from mentors and other health and allied professionals, competency in identifying clinical problems, the ability to search the literature for research, critical skills to interpret research findings, and willingness and ability to design and participate in research. Levels of clinical inquiry include:

- Level 1: This nurse recognizes problems and seeks advice, follows industry standards and guidelines, and seeks further knowledge.
- Level 3: This nurse questions industry standards and guidelines as well as current practice and utilizes research and education to improve patient care.
- Level 5: This nurse is able to deviate from industry standards and guidelines when necessary for individual patients and utilizes literature review and clinical research to gain knowledge, establish new practices, and improve patient care.

### Evidence-based guidelines

Steps to evidence-based practice guidelines include:

- ***Focus on the topic/methodology:*** This includes outlining possible interventions/treatments for review, choosing patient populations and settings and determining significant outcomes. Search boundaries (such as types of journals, types of studies, and dates of studies) should be determined.
- ***Evidence review:*** This includes review of literature, critical analysis of studies, and summarizing of results, including pooled meta-analysis.
- ***Expert judgment:*** Recommendations based on personal experience from a number of experts may be utilized, especially if there is inadequate evidence based on review, but this subjective evidence should be explicated and acknowledged.
- ***Policy considerations:*** This includes cost-effectiveness, access to care, insurance

Copyright © Mometrix Media. You have been licensed one copy of this document for personal use only. Any other reproduction or redistribution is strictly prohibited. All rights reserved.

coverage, availability of qualified staff, and legal implications.

- **Policy:** A written policy must be completed with recommendations. Common practice is to utilize letter guidelines, with "A" the most highly recommended, usually based the quality of supporting evidence.
- **Review:** The completed policy should be submitted to peers for review and comments before instituting the policy.

## Developing clinical/critical pathways

Clinical/critical pathway development is done by those involved in direct patient care. The pathway should require no additional staffing and cover the entire scope of an illness. Steps include:

- Selection of the patient group and diagnosis, procedures, or conditions, based on analysis of data and observations of wide variance in approach to treatment and prioritizing organization and patient needs.
- Creation of an interdisciplinary team of those involved in the process of care, including physicians to develop pathway.
- Analysis of data includes literature review and study of best practices to identify opportunities for quality improvement.
- Identification of all categories of care, such as nutrition, medications, nursing.
- Discussion, reaching consensus.
- Identifying the levels of care and number of days to be covered by the pathway.
- Pilot testing and redesigning steps as indicated.
- Educating staff about standards.
- Monitoring and tracking variances in order to improve pathways.

## Basic research concepts

The nurse must be taught to understand the process of critical analysis and know how to conduct a survey of the literature. Basic research concepts include:

- **Survey of valid sources:** Information from a juried journal and an anonymous website or

personal website are very different sources, and evaluating what constitutes a valid source of data is critical.
- **Evaluation of internal and external validity:** Internal validity shows a cause and effect relationship between 2 variables, with the cause occurring before the effect and no intervening variable. External validity occurs when results hold true in different environments and circumstances with different populations.
- **Sample selection and sample size:** Selection and size can have a huge impact on the results. A sample that is too small may lack both internal and external validity. Selection may be so narrowly focused that the results can't be generalized to other groups.

Reading research articles:
There are a number of steps to critical reading to evaluate research:

- **Consider the source** of the material. If it is in the popular press, it may have little validity compared to something published in a juried journal.
- **Review the author's credentials** to determine if a person is an expert in the field of study.
- **Determine thesis**, or the central claim of the research. It should be clearly stated.
- **Examine the organization** of the article, whether it is based on a particular theory, and the type of methodology used.
- **Review the evidence** to determine how it is used to support the main points. Look for statistical evidence and sample size to determine if the findings have wide applicability.
- **Evaluate** the overall article to determine if the information seems credible and useful and should be communicated to the administration and/or staff.

Validity:
Many research studies are most concerned with internal validity, i.e., adequate unbiased data properly collected and analyzed within the population studied, but studies that determine

Copyright © Mometrix Media. You have been licensed one copy of this document for personal use only. Any other reproduction or redistribution is strictly prohibited. All rights reserved.

the efficacy of procedures or treatments, for example, should have external validity as well; that is, the results should be generalizable (true) for similar populations. Replication of the study with different subjects, researchers, and under different circumstances should produce similar results. For various reasons, some people may be excluded from a study, so instead of randomized subjects, the subjects may be highly selected. When data are compared with another population in which there is less or more selection, the results may be different. The selection of subjects, in this case, would interfere with external validity. Part of the design of a study should include considerations of whether or not it should have external validity or whether there is value for the institution based solely on internal validation.

Selection bias:
Selection bias occurs when the method of selecting subjects results in a cohort that is not representative of the target population because of inherent error in design. For example, if all infants who develop urinary infections are evaluated per urine culture and sensitivities for microbial resistance, but only those infants with clinically-evident infections are included, a number of patients with sub-clinical infections may be missed, skewing the results. Selection bias is only a concern when participants in studies are specifically chosen. Many surveillance studies do not involve selection of subjects.

Information bias:
Information bias occurs when there are errors in classification, so an estimate of association is incorrect. Non-differential misclassification occurs when there is similar misclassification of disease or exposure among both those who are diseased/exposed and those who are not. Differential misclassification occurs when there is a differing misclassification of disease or exposure among both those who are diseased/exposed and those who are not.

Qualitative and quantitative data:
Both qualitative and quantitative data are used for analysis, but the focus is quite different:

- **Qualitative data**: Data are described verbally or graphically, and the results are subjective, depending upon observers to provide information. Interviews may be used as a tool to gather information, and the researcher's interpretation of data is important. Gathering this type of data can be time-intensive, and it cannot usually be generalized to a larger population. This type of information gathering is often useful at the beginning of the design process for data collection.
- **Quantitative data**: Data are described in terms of numbers within a statistical format. This type of information gathering is done after the design of data collection is outlined, usually in later stages. Tools may include surveys, questionnaires, or other methods of obtaining numerical data. The researcher's role is objective.

## Hypothesis

A hypothesis should be generated about the probable cause of the disease/infection based on the information available in laboratory and medical records, epidemiologic study, literature review, and expert opinion. A hypothesis, for example, should include the infective agent, the likely source, and the mode of transmission: "Wound infections with *Staphylococcus aureus* were caused by reuse and inadequate sterilization of single-use irrigation syringes used during wound care in the ICU." Hypothesis testing includes data analysis, laboratory findings, and outcomes of environmental testing. It usually includes *case control studies*, with 2-4 controls picked for each case of infection. They may be matched according to age, sex, or other characteristics, but they are not infected at the time they are picked for the study. *Cohort studies,* whose controls are picked based on having or lacking exposure, may also be instituted. If the hypothesis cannot be supported, then a new hypothesis or different testing methods may be necessary.

*Copyright © Mometrix Media. You have been licensed one copy of this document for personal use only. Any other reproduction or redistribution is strictly prohibited. All rights reserved.*

## Outcomes evaluation

Outcomes evaluation is an important component of evidence-based practice, which involves both internal and external research. All treatments are subjected to review to determine if they produce positive outcomes, and policies and protocols for outcomes evaluation should be in place. Outcomes evaluation includes the following:

- **Monitoring** over the course of treatment involves careful observation and record keeping that notes progress, with supporting laboratory and radiographic evidence, as indicated by the condition and treatment.
- **Evaluating** results includes reviewing records, as well as current research, to determine if outcomes are within acceptable parameters.
- **Sustaining** involves continuing treatment but continuing to monitor and evaluate.
- **Improving** means to continue the treatment but with additions or modifications in order to improve outcomes.
- **Replacing** the treatment with a different treatment must be done, if outcomes evaluation indicates that current treatment is ineffective.

## *Facilitation of Learning*

### Facilitation of learning

In the ACCN synergy model, facilitation of learning is the ability to facilitate learning by patient and family/caregivers as well as other health and allied professionals and community members. Facilitation of learning requires needs assessment and preparation of content that is suited for the receiver, regarding its delivery and content. Levels of facilitation of learning include:

- Level 1: This nurse is able to deliver planned educational content that is disease specific but does not have the ability to assess patient readiness to learn or ability level. The patient/family is considered a passive recipient of knowledge.
- Level 3: This nurse is able to individualize treatment according to patient/family needs and has an understanding of different methods of teaching and learning styles. The patient's needs are considered in planning.
- Level 5: This nurse has an excellent understanding of teaching methods, learning styles, and assessment for learning readiness; the nurse develops an educational plan in cooperation and collaboration with patients, families, health, and allied health professionals.

### Development of education plan

Once a topic for performance improvement education has been chosen, then goals, measurable objectives with strategies, and lesson plans must be developed. A class should stay focused on one area rather than trying to cover many things. For example:

| Goal | Increase compliance with hand hygiene standards in ICU. |
|---|---|
| **Objectives** | Develop a series of posters and fliers by June 1. Observe 100% compliance with hand hygiene standards at 2 weeks, 1-month, and 2-month intervals after training is completed. |
| **Strategies** | Conduct 4 classes at different times over a 1-week period, May 25-31. Place posters in all nursing units, staff rooms, and utility rooms by January 3. Develop PowerPoint presentation for class and Intranet/Internet for access by all staff by May 25. Utilize hand washing kits. |
| **Lesson plans** | Discussion period: Why do we need 100% compliance? PowerPoint: The case for hand hygiene. Discussion: What did you learn? Demonstration and activities to show effectiveness. Hand washing technique. |

Copyright © Mometrix Media. You have been licensed one copy of this document for personal use only. Any other reproduction or redistribution is strictly prohibited. All rights reserved.

## Approaches to teaching

There are many approaches to teaching, and the nurse-educator must prepare, present, and coordinate a wide range of educational workshops, lectures, discussions, and one-on-one instructions on any chosen topic. All types of classes will be needed, depending upon the purpose and material:

- **Educational workshops** are usually conducted with small groups, allowing for maximal participation and are especially good for demonstrations and practice sessions.
- **Lectures** are often used for more academic or detailed information that may include questions and answers but limits discussion. An effective lecture should include some audiovisual support.
- **Discussions** are best with small groups so that people can actively participate. This is a good for problem solving.
- **One-on-one instruction** is especially helpful for targeted instruction in procedures for individuals.
- **Computer/Internet modules** are good for independent learners.

Participants should be asked to evaluate the presentations by completing surveys or making suggestions, but ultimately the program is evaluated in terms of patient outcomes.

Videos:
Videos are a useful adjunct to teaching as they reduce the time needed for one-on-one instruction (increasing cost-effectiveness). Passive presentation of videos, such as in the waiting area, has little value, but focused viewing in which the nurse discusses the purpose of the video presentation prior to viewing and then is available for discussion afterwards can be very effective. Patients and/or families are often nervous about learning patient care and are unsure of their abilities, so they may not focus completely when the nurse is presenting information. Allowing the patients/families to watch a video demonstration or explanation first and allowing them to stop or review the video

presentation can help them grasp the fundamentals before they have to apply them, relieving some of the anxiety they may be experiencing. Videos are much more effective than written materials for those with low literacy or limited English skills. The nurse should always be available to answer questions and discuss the material after the patients/families finish viewing.

Reading materials:
Studies have indicated that learning is more effective if oral presentations and/or demonstrations are supplemented with reading materials, such as handouts. Readability (the grade level of material) is a concern because many patients and families have limited English skills or low literacy, and it is difficult for the nurse to assess a person's reading level. The average American reads effectively at the 6th to 8th grade level (regardless of education achieved), but many health education materials have a much higher readability level. Additionally, research indicates that even people with much higher reading skills learn medical and health information most effectively when the material is presented at the 6th to 8th grade readability level. Therefore, patient education materials (and consent forms) should not be written at higher than the 6th to 8th grade level. Readability index calculators are available on the Internet to give an approximation of grade level and difficulty for those preparing materials but who are without expertise in teaching reading.

## Educating staff on changes

Changes in policies, procedures, or working standards are common, and the quality professional is responsible for educating the staff about changes related to processes and for communicating these to the staff in an effective and timely manner:

- **Policies** are usually changed after a period of discussion and review by the administration and staff, so all staff should be made aware of the policies under discussion. Preliminary information should be disseminated to the

*Copyright © Mometrix Media. You have been licensed one copy of this document for personal use only. Any other reproduction or redistribution is strictly prohibited. All rights reserved.*

staff regarding the issue during meetings or through printed notices.

- **Procedures** may be changed to increase efficiency or improve patient safety, often as the result of surveillance and data about outcomes. Procedural changes are best communicated in workshops with demonstrations. Posters and handouts should be available as well.
- **Working standards** are often changed because of regulatory or accrediting requirements, and this information should be covered extensively in a variety of different ways: discussions, workshops, and handouts so that the implications are clearly understood.

## Learning styles

Not all people are aware of their preferred learning style. A range of teaching materials/methods that relates to all 3 learning preferences—visual, auditory, kinesthetic—(and appropriate for different ages) should be available. Part of the assessment for teaching involves choosing the right approach based on observation and feedback. Often presenting learners with different options gives a clue to their preferred learning style. Some people have a combined learning style:

| *Visual learners* | Learn best by seeing and reading: Provide written directions, picture guides, or demonstrate procedures. Use charts and diagrams. Provide photos and videos. |
|---|---|
| *Auditory learners* | Learn best by listening and talking: Explain procedures while demonstrating and have learner repeat. Plan extra time to discuss and answer questions. Provide audiotapes. |
| *Kinesthetic learners* | Learn best by handling, doing, and practicing: Provide hands-on experience throughout teaching. Encourage handling of |

| | supplies/equipment. Allow learner to demonstrate. Minimize instructions and allow person to explore equipment and procedures. |
|---|---|

## Adult learning

Adults have a wealth of life and/or employment experiences. Their attitudes toward education may vary considerably. There are, however, some principles of adult learning and typical characteristics of adult learners that an instructor should consider when planning strategies for teaching parents, families, or staff:

| *Practical and goal-oriented* | Provide overviews or summaries and examples. Use collaborative discussions with problem-solving exercises. Remain organized with the goal in mind. |
|---|---|
| *Self-directed* | Provide active involvement, asking for input. Allow different options toward achieving the goal. Give them responsibilities. |
| *Knowledgeable* | Show respect for their life experiences/education. Validate their knowledge and ask for feedback. Relate new material to information with which they are familiar. |
| *Relevancy-oriented* | Explain how information will be applied. Clearly identify objectives. |
| *Motivated* | Provide certificates of professional advancement and/or continuing education credit for staff, when possible. |

## Bloom's taxonomy

Bloom's taxonomy outlines behaviors that are necessary for learning, and this can apply to healthcare. The theory describes 3 types of learning:

- **Cognitive** (Learning and gaining intellectual skills to master 6 categories of effective learning.):

*Copyright © Mometrix Media. You have been licensed one copy of this document for personal use only. Any other reproduction or redistribution is strictly prohibited. All rights reserved.*

- o *Knowledge, Comprehension, Application, Analysis, Synthesis, Evaluation.*
- **Affective** (Recognizing 5 categories of feelings and values from simple to complex. This is slower to achieve than cognitive learning.)
  - o *Receiving phenomena:* Accepting need to learn.
  - o *Responding to phenomena:* Taking active part in care.
  - o *Valuing:* Understanding value of becoming independent in care.
  - o *Organizing values:* Understanding how surgery/treatment has improved life.
  - o *Internalizing values:* Accepting condition as part of life, being consistent and self-reliant.
- **Psychomotor** (Mastering motor skills necessary for independence. This follows a progression from simple to complex.)
  - o *Perception*: Uses sensory information to learn tasks.
  - o *Set:* Shows willingness to perform tasks.
  - o *Guided response:* Follows directions.
  - o *Mechanism:* Does specific tasks.
  - o *Complex overt response:* Displays competence in self-care.
  - o *Adaptation:* Modifies procedures as needed.
  - o *Origination:* Creatively deals with problems.

## Behavior modification

Education, like all interventions, must be evaluated for effectiveness. Two determinants of effectiveness include

- **Behavior modification** involves thorough observation and measurement, identifying behavior that needs to be changed and then planning and instituting interventions to modify that behavior. An ACNP can use a variety of techniques, including demonstrations of appropriate behavior, reinforcement, and monitoring until a new behavior is adopted consistently. This is especially important when longstanding procedures and habits of behavior are changed.

- **Compliance rates** are often determined by observation, which should be done at intervals and on multiple occasions, but with patients, this may depend on self-reports. Outcomes are another measure of compliance; that is, if education is intended to improve patient health and reduce risk factors and that occurs, it is a good indication that there is compliance. Compliance rates are calculated by determining the number of events/procedures and degree of compliance.

## Learner outcomes

When the quality professional plans an educational offering, whether it is a class, an online module, a workshop, or educational materials, the professional should identify learner outcomes, which should be conveyed to the learners from the very beginning so that they are aware of the expectations. The subject matter of the educational material and the learner outcomes should be directly related. For example, if the quality professional is giving a class on decontamination of the environment, then a learner outcome might be: "Identify the difference between disinfectants and antiseptics." There may be one or multiple learner outcomes, but part of the assessment at the end of the learning experience should be to determine if, in fact, the learner outcomes have been achieved. A survey of whether or not the learners felt that they had achieved the learner outcomes can give valuable feedback and guidance to the quality professional.

## Patient/family education

Both one-on-one instruction and group instruction have a place in patient/family education.

- **One-on-one instruction** is the most costly for an institution because it is time intensive. However, it allows the patient and family more interaction with the nurse-instructor and allows them to have more control over the process by asking questions or having the instructor repeat explanations or

*Copyright © Mometrix Media. You have been licensed one copy of this document for personal use only. Any other reproduction or redistribution is strictly prohibited. All rights reserved.*

demonstrations. One-on-one instruction is especially valuable when patients and families must learn particular skills, such as managing dialysis, or if confidentiality is important.

- **Group instruction** is the less costly because the needs of a number of people can be met at one time. Group presentations are more planned and usually scheduled for a particular time period (an hour, for example), so patients and families have less control. Questioning is usually more limited and may be done only at the end. Group instruction allows patients/families with similar health problems to interact. Group instruction is especially useful for general types of instruction, such as managing diet or other lifestyle issues.

## Readiness to learn

**Readiness to learn** includes:

- **Mental/emotional status:** The support system and motivation may impact readiness. Anxiety, fear, or depression about condition can make learning very difficult because the patient/family cannot focus on learning, so the nurse must spend time to reassure the patient/family and wait until they are emotionally more receptive.
- **Knowledge/education:** The knowledge base of the patient/family, their cognitive ability, and their learning styles all affect their readiness to learn. The nurse should always begin by assessing what knowledge the patient/family already has about the disease, condition, or treatment and then build from that base. People with little medical experience may lack knowledge of basic medical terminology, interfering with their ability and readiness to learn.

Copyright © Mometrix Media. You have been licensed one copy of this document for personal use only. Any other reproduction or redistribution is strictly prohibited. All rights reserved.

# Practice Test

## Practice Questions

1. A 58-year-old male with a history of alcohol abuse is a heavy smoker. He complains of pain in his chest in the afternoons when he is sitting and watching TV. ECG shows elevation of ST segments. The most likely diagnosis is:
   a. Unstable angina.
   b. Variant/Prinzmetal's angina.
   c. Stable angina.
   d. Gastroesophageal reflux disease.

2. Metabolic syndrome is characterized by:
   a. Abdominal obesity, decreased triglyceride level, increased HDL level, and hypertension.
   b. Hypertension, abdominal obesity, and increased HDL level.
   c. Abdominal obesity, increased triglyceride level, decreased HDL level, and increased fasting blood glucose level.
   d. Hypotension, decreased fasting blood glucose level, increased triglyceride level, and decreased HDL level.

3. Parenteral nutrition with a total nutrient admixture that includes lipids has been ordered for a burn patient for administration throughout a 24-hour period. When preparing to administer the solution, the nurse observes that the oil has separated, forming an obvious layer. Which of the following options is the correct action to take?
   a. Administer the solution, as oil separation is normal.
   b. Mix the solution by shaking the bag until no oil separation is noticeable.
   c. Discard the solution.
   d. Return the solution to the pharmacy for the addition of added emulsifier.

4. A 30-year-old patient complains of post-operative pain at 8 on a 1-to-10 scale 12 hours after surgery, but is not moaning, grimacing, or exhibiting any standard physical signs of pain.

The patient last received pain medication 6 hours earlier, and has orders for morphine every 4 hours as needed and ibuprofen every 6 hours as needed. Which is the most appropriate action?
   a. Administer ibuprofen.
   b. Administer morphine.
   c. Administer ibuprofen, and if the patient does not feel relief after one hour post-dose, then administer morphine.
   d. Question present family members about the patient's pain tolerance before making a decision.

5. Q-wave myocardial infarction is characterized by:
   a. ST-T wave changes with ST depression that reverses within a few days.
   b. Small infarct size-due to spontaneous reperfusion.
   c. Peak CK levels in 12 to 13 hours.
   d. Complete coronary occlusion in 80% to 90% of patients.

6. A nursing team leader delegates a task to an unlicensed assistive member of the personnel. Who is responsible for patient outcomes?
   a. The unlicensed person who completes the task
   b. Both the team leader and the unlicensed person who completes the task
   c. The team leader who delegates the task
   d. The administrative staff

7. A patient with acute lung injury has crackling râles, tachypnea, and cyanosis. Oxygen therapy is instituted to maintain oxygen saturation at:
   a. ≥85%
   b. >90%
   c. >95%
   d. ≥98%

8. The normal blood, urea, nitrogen (BUN)/creatinine ratio is:
   a. 5:1
   b. 8:1
   c. 10:1
   d. 20:1

*Copyright © Mometrix Media. You have been licensed one copy of this document for personal use only. Any other reproduction or redistribution is strictly prohibited. All rights reserved.*

9. A myocardial infarction usually causes damage to the myocardium, progressing from the endocardium to the epicardium. The first stage in myocardial damage is:
- a. Formation of zone of ischemia
- b. Formation of zone of necrosis
- c. Formation of zone of injury
- d. Decreased perfusion from hypotension

10. A patient presents with pulmonary edema characterized by tachypnea, tachycardia, hypertension, cough, fever, and cough with frothy sanguineous sputum. What initial treatments are most common?
- a. Oxygen, nitroglycerine, loop diuretics (furosemide), and morphine
- b. Oxygen, thiazide diuretics, and ACE inhibitors
- c. Oxygen and thiazide diuretics
- d. Oxygen, morphine, and calcium channel blockers

11. A 70-year-old female patient with a leg wound is being treated with negative-pressure wound therapy using a vacuum-assisted closure system. The most appropriate non-adherent porous foam for a wound that is painful and has tunneling is:
- a. Polyurethane (hydrophobic, repelling moisture)
- b. Polyvinyl (hydrophilic)
- c. Either polyurethane or polyvinyl
- d. Neither polyurethane nor polyvinyl

12. A patient presents with the classic signs of a myocardial infarction, including crushing chest pain, radiating to the arms and neck, palpitations, pallor, and dyspnea. The patient most likely to experience these symptoms is:
- a. A 60-year-old male
- b. A 52-year-old male with type 1 diabetes and neuropathy
- c. A 54-year-old female
- d. An 86-year-old female with Alzheimer's disease

13. The Health Insurance Portability and Accountability Act (HIPAA) regulates:
- a. The transfer of patients from one facility to another
- b. Clinical trials
- c. Workplace safety
- d. The rights of the individual related to privacy of health information

14. A 24-year-old female developed hepatitis after eating contaminated food in a restaurant. Which form of hepatitis does she probably have?
- a. Fulminant hepatitis
- b. Hepatitis A
- c. Hepatitis B
- d. Hepatitis C

15. A 48-year-old female patient has terminal ovarian cancer but states she believes her doctor has misdiagnosed her and that she wants to see a different doctor. Which stage of Elisabeth Kübler-Ross's stages of grief (death and dying) is she likely experiencing?
- a. Anger
- b. Denial
- c. Depression
- d. Bargaining

16. A 76-year-old female with advanced Parkinson's disease develops cough, dyspnea, and wheezing. Râles are noted in the right lung, and a chest radiograph shows infiltrates in the right lung below the right bronchus. The most likely diagnosis is:
- a. Foreign-body aspiration
- b. Pulmonary edema
- c. Pneumonia
- d. Pulmonary embolism

17. A patient who experienced an episode of severe chest pain and weakness 4 days earlier is undergoing diagnostic tests. Which test would provide the most accurate information to diagnose an MI after 4 days?
- a. ECG
- b. Creatinine-kinase and isoenzyme (CK-MB)
- c. Myoglobin
- d. Troponin and its isomers (C, I, and T)

*Copyright © Mometrix Media. You have been licensed one copy of this document for personal use only. Any other reproduction or redistribution is strictly prohibited. All rights reserved.*

18. A patient is admitted to the unit after vomiting excessively for 4 days at home. The patient's serum pH is elevated, $PCO_2$ is relatively normal, and the urine pH is >6. The patient is dizzy, confused and is exhibiting tremors, seizures, tingling, tachycardia, arrhythmias, and hypoventilation. The patient is most likely exhibiting symptoms of:
   a. Respiratory alkalosis
   b. Metabolic alkalosis
   c. Respiratory acidosis
   d. Metabolic acidosis

19. A patient receiving chemotherapy for cancer has developed malnutrition and is receiving parenteral feedings, but the patient has developed abdominal discomfort, nausea, and diarrhea with resultant dehydration, hypotension, and tachycardia. What is the most appropriate action?
   a. Reduce the osmolality of the solution and then increase slowly
   b. Check tube placement
   c. Lower glucose content of solution
   d. Keep head of the bed elevated at all times

20. Janeway lesions, splinter hemorrhages, mucosal petechiae, and Roth's spots are most characteristic of which of the following cardiac disorders?
   a. Myocardial infarction
   b. Endocarditis
   c. Myocarditis
   d. Pericarditis

21. A patient with gastroenteritis has been diagnosed with severe dehydration (>15% fluid loss). Typical symptoms include:
   a. Dry mouth and increased thirst
   b. Dizziness, lethargy, reduced skin turgor, and orthostatic hypotension
   c. Resting hypotension, confusion, tachycardia, and oliguria
   d. Hypotension and anuria in addition to other symptoms

22. Neurogenic shock is often characterized by:
   a. Tachycardia
   b. Diaphoresis

   c. Bradycardia
   d. Hyperthermia

23. Which of the following is an example of therapeutic communication?
   a. "Don't worry. Everything will be fine."
   b. "You should listen to your doctor."
   c. "Why are you upset?"
   d. "Is there anything you'd like to discuss?"

24. A patient with chronic ventilatory failure has $PCO_2$ >50 and pH <7.35 with dyspnea, cardiac arrhythmias, confusion, hyperkalemia, and hypotension: These findings are consistent with:
   a. Respiratory acidosis
   b. Respiratory alkalosis
   c. Metabolic acidosis
   d. Metabolic alkalosis

25. The best time to initiate conflict resolution is:
   a. When those in conflict have had time to resolve their differences
   b. When conflict interferes with function
   c. When those involved ask for conflict resolution
   d. At the initial emergence of conflict

26. A 75-year-old male patient had a stroke two months ago. He has left-sided paresis, left visual field defect, and impaired motor skills. His language skills are intact, but he behaves impulsively, has difficulty following directions, and suffers from short-term memory loss. His stroke most likely occurred in the:
   a. Right hemisphere
   b. Left hemisphere
   c. Brain stem
   d. Cerebellum

27. Which of the following disorders is medically treated with aspirin or other anti-inflammatory drugs, such as ibuprofen?
   a. Endocarditis
   b. Myocarditis
   c. Pericarditis
   d. Angina

28. The "5 rights of delegation" include:

*Copyright © Mometrix Media. You have been licensed one copy of this document for personal use only. Any other reproduction or redistribution is strictly prohibited. All rights reserved.*

a. Right time, right place, right person, right direction, and right evaluation.

b. Right person, right place, right time, right assignment, and right supervision.

c. Right task, right time, right circumstance, right place, and right supervision.

d. Right task, right circumstance, right person, right direction, and right supervision.

29. A 40-year-old female with type 1 diabetes presents with hyperventilation, dehydration with diuresis and increased thirst, and cardiac arrhythmias. Initial treatment will probably include:

a. (Hyperstat®) to inhibit release of insulin

b. (Glucose) for hypoglycemia and electrolyte therapy only for dehydration

c. Insulin therapy for ketoacidosis and fluid (non-glucose) and electrolyte replacement

d. Intravenous glucose solution for hypoglycemia

30. Which of the following tests is the most accurate in the diagnosis of myocarditis?

a. Polymerase chain reaction (PCR) of biopsy specimen

b. Echocardiogram

c. Electrocardiogram

d. Cardiac catheterization and biopsy

31. A patient is admitted with an acute exacerbation of COPD. Under which of the following circumstances is theophylline indicated?

a. As first-line treatment to relieve dyspnea

b. After achieving no response from short-acting bronchodilators.

c. Before the administration of corticosteroids only

d. After no response is achieved from short-acting and/or long-acting bronchodilators or corticosteroids

32. During the interdisciplinary team meeting, the leader stresses the importance of following the rules of the organization exactly. Of which style of leadershipis this an example?

a. Autocratic

b. Consultative

c. Participatory

d. Bureaucratic

33. A patient is scheduled for surgery for a defective aortic valve. Which of the following procedures is probably NOT indicated?

a. Balloon valvuloplasty

b. Ross procedure

c. Aortic homograft

d. Aortic valve replacement

34. In evaluating outcomes of nutritional intervention for a patient with type 2 diabetes mellitus and a fasting blood sugar level of 130 mg/dL three months ago, which lab result best indicates dietary compliance?

a. Fasting blood sugar of 106 mg/dL

b. Hemoglobin A1C of 6.6%

c. Hemoglobin A1C of 5.5%

d. Fasting blood sugar of 150 mg/dL

35. A 62-year-old male with pancreatitis has received narcotic medications to reduce pain. He has increased nausea and vomiting and his abdomen becomes distended and uncomfortable. He has an absence of flatulence and bowel sounds. The most likely diagnosis is:

a. Bowel obstruction

b. Paralytic ileus

c. Bowel infarction

d. Short gut syndrome

36. A thoracentesis is often done with the patient sitting in the upright position. An alternate position for those unable to sit upright is:

a. Lying on the affected side with the head of the bed flat

b. Lying on the affected side with the head of the bed elevated to 30° to 45°

c. Lying on the opposite side with the head of the bed elevated to 20°

d. Lying on the opposite side with the head of the bed elevated to 30° to 45°

37. According to the ANA Nursing Code of Ethics, nurses must support a patient's autonomy and self-determination. If a 24 year-old Asian female

*Copyright © Mometrix Media. You have been licensed one copy of this document for personal use only. Any other reproduction or redistribution is strictly prohibited. All rights reserved.*

patient states a treatment preference but plans to leave the decision to family members, the nurse should:

    a. Try to convince the patient to assert herself

    b. Recognize that cultural values regarding individualism vary and respect the patient's right to be guided by family

    c. Tell the family that the patient should be the one to make the decision

    d. Ask the ethics committee to intervene

38. A patient is receiving daily warfarin after treatment for atrial fibrillation. Which of the following may interfere with the drug's effectiveness?

    a. One 8-ounce glass of red wine daily

    b. Caffeinated beverages

    c. A daily multivitamin

    d. Milk products

39. A postoperative patient develops disseminated intravascular coagulation (DIC) with bleeding from operative and puncture sites, GI bleeding with distention and bloody diarrhea, petechiae, purpura, hypotension, and acute symptoms of shock. Expected laboratory findings include:

    a. Decreased prothrombin and partial prothrombin times and increased platelet count and fibrinogen

    b. Prolonged prothrombin and partial prothrombin times and increased platelet count and decreased fibrinogen

    c. Prolonged prothrombin and partial prothrombin times and decreased platelet count and fibrinogen

    d. Decreased prothrombin and partial prothrombin times and decreased platelet count and increased fibrinogen

40. A 40-year-old female with terminal lung cancer develops an acute sudden change in consciousness, characterized by fluctuating symptoms of disorientation, confusion, audiovisual hallucinations, sleep disturbance, and memory disturbance. The most likely diagnosis is:

    a. Delirium

    b. Metastasis

    c. Severe malnutrition

    d. Electrolyte imbalance

41. A team leader is preparing for a team meeting. What is the best approach to an agenda?

    a. Prepare only a general agenda and add topics as needed during the meeting

    b. Prepare a detailed agenda of topics for discussion

    c. Ask for topics of discussion at the beginning of the meeting and prioritize and create an agenda at that time

    d. Prepare no agenda but have a free discussion

42. A patient is being treated for renal disease and exhibits the following: ventricular arrhythmia with increasing ECG changes, weakness with ascending paralysis and hyperreflexia, diarrhea, and increasing confusion. The patient is most likely suffering from:

    a. Hyperkalemia

    b. Hypokalemia

    c. Hypocalcemia

    d. Hypercalcemia

43. A 68-year-old male is 4 hours postoperative after percutaneous transluminal coronary angioplasty (PTCA) and complains of pain in the flank area. He is restless, tachycardic, and hypotensive, and his hemoglobin and hematocrit have dropped. Which of the following nursing actions is correct?

    a. Keep the head of the bed flat and apply pressure at the sheath site to stop bleeding

    b. Notify a physician immediately and anticipate ultrasound-guided compression and possible surgery to close fistula

    c. Notify a physician immediately and anticipate anticoagulation or thrombolytic therapy.

    d. Notify a physician immediately, stop anticoagulation therapy, and anticipate need for intravenous fluids and/or blood.

*Copyright © Mometrix Media. You have been licensed one copy of this document for personal use only. Any other reproduction or redistribution is strictly prohibited. All rights reserved.*

44. After a spinal tap, the patient complains of severe headache, visual disturbances, and nausea. An autologous blood patch may be injected epidurally near the puncture site in order to:

    a. Prevent infection
    b. Relieve local pain at the puncture site
    c. Plug the puncture hole in the dura
    d. Reduce edema at the puncture site

45. A 30-year-old male complains of frequent nosebleeds, abdominal pain, and nausea. He has burns on his fingers and a slight cough but no needle marks, and his pupils are constricted. He sniffs repeatedly because of nasal irritation. He has a slight fever and tachycardia, and he is malnourished. What substance has he likely been abusing?

    a. Cocaine
    b. Heroin
    c. Marijuana
    d Methadone

46. A 35-year-old female recovering from chest surgery has a chest tube to a water seal (wet suction). In which chamber(s) is sterile fluid instilled?

    a. Into the first (collection) and third (wet suction) chambers
    b. Into the water seal chamber only to the 2 cm level
    c. Into the middle water seal chamber only
    d. Into the middle water seal and the third (wet suction) chambers

47. Which of the following increases the risk of ReoPro®-induced coagulopathy and is a contraindication for use?

    a. Previous stroke within three years
    b. Platelet count of 110,000 mm³
    c. Recent warfarin therapy
    d. History of angina

48. The nurse should identify learner outcomes as part of the plan for an educational offering. An example of a learner outcome for teaching diabetics about insulin reaction is:

    a. Identifying the different types of insulin
    b. Listing and describing the symptoms of insulin reaction

    c. Identifying foods high in carbohydrates
    d. Explaining the difference between type 1 and type 2 diabetes

49. A patient recovering from a coronary artery bypass graft (CABG) develops disorientation that progresses to agitation, hallucinations, and paranoia on the third postoperative day. Which of the following complications of cardiac surgery does this most likely suggest?

    a. Cardiac ischemia
    b. Stroke
    c. Pulmonary embolism
    d. Postcardiotomy delirium

50. Oxygen concentration with nasal cannula delivery ranges from:

    a. 24% to 44%
    b. 50% to 64%
    c. 70% to 84%
    d. 90% to 100%

51. Which of the following is NOT a barrier to systems thinking?

    a. A holistic view of interrelationships within the organization
    b. Identification with role rather than purpose
    c. Reliance on past experience
    d. Feelings of victimization

52. Pulse oximetry is continually monitored after cardiac surgery. Arterial oxygen saturation ($SPO_2$) levels should be maintained at:

    a. ≥90%
    b. ≥92%
    c. ≥95%
    d. ≥98%

53. An 80-year-old female presents with a small pneumothorax upon the administration of a chest radiograph, but is not in acute distress. Which of the following treatments is the most appropriate?

    a. Chest-tube thoracostomy with underwater seal drainage
    b. Immediate needle decompression and chest-tube thoracostomy
    c. Catheter aspiration

Copyright © Mometrix Media. You have been licensed one copy of this document for personal use only. Any other reproduction or redistribution is strictly prohibited. All rights reserved.

d. Administration of oxygen at 3 to 4 L/min and observation for 3 to 6 hours and repeat chest x-ray to monitor change

54. When evaluating cardiac output in a normal heart, a decrease in heart rate should cause the stroke volume to:
    a. Increase
    b. Decrease
    c. Remain unchanged
    d. Vary

55. The nurse is teaching a patient to manage tracheostomy care. The nurse has prepared written directions and a video, but the patient ignores them and picks up the pieces of equipment and looks at each part, trying to figure it out. The patient's learning style is most likely:
    a. Auditory
    b. Visual
    c. Kinesthetic
    d. Mixed

56. A 70-year-old male with chronic cirrhosis and hepatic failure has developed portal hypertension. Which of the following is the most common complication of portal hypertension?
    a. Jaundice
    b. Blockage of the bile duct
    c. Hemorrhage of esophageal varices
    d. Abdominal distention

57. A patient experiences diuresis and dehydration after cardiac surgery, causing his preload to:
    a. Increase
    b. Decrease
    c. Remain unaffected
    d. Rapidly fluctuate

58. Acute renal failure resulting from sepsis is caused by:
    a. Hypoperfusion and decreased glomerular filtration rate (GFR)
    b. Hemolysis with the broken down hemoglobin concentrating and precipitating in tubules
    c. Damage to glomeruli or kidney tubules

d. Increased pressure in tubules and decreased GFR

59. A patient is one-day postoperative following surgery for peripheral vascular disease. She is increasingly restless and develops a low-grade fever, hiccoughs, dyspnea, cough, tachycardia, and chest pain. Which of the following diagnoses is the most likely?
    a. Atelectasis
    b. Myocardial infarction
    c. Pulmonary embolism
    d. Pneumonitis

60. Thoracic electrical bioimpedence monitoring with 4 sets of bioimpedence electrodes and 3 ECG electrodes is used to evaluate hemodynamic status of a postsurgical cardiac patient. Where are the bioimpedence electrodes placed?
    a. One set on the arms, one set on the legs, and one set on the sides of the chest.
    b. Two sets bilaterally at the base of the neck and two sets on each side of the chest.
    c. One set on the legs and three sets on each side of the chest.
    d. One set on the arms, one set bilaterally at the base of the neck, and two sets on each side of the chest.

61. A 50-year-old man dying of cardiovascular disease is Catholic and asks to take final communion even though it is 2:00 AM. The nurse should:
    a. Contact the patient's priest or a priest on call for the institution and ask him to come right away
    b. Tell the patient that no priest is available
    c. Ask the patient if he would be willing to see the Protestant chaplain who is on call
    d. Tell the patient the priest will be called at 7:00 AM

62. A 52-year-old female with a history of bipolar disease is one-day post-operative following a hip replacement. The patient slept only one or two hours during the night and is speaking rapidly, throwing her belongings at the nurses, and insisting she is going to leave the hospital against medical advice. The nurse should notify:

Copyright © Mometrix Media. You have been licensed one copy of this document for personal use only. Any other reproduction or redistribution is strictly prohibited. All rights reserved.

a. The mental health crisis team
b. Social services
c. A home health agency
d. The patient's husband

63. If all patients who develop urinary infections are evaluated per urine culture and sensitivities for microbial resistance, but only those with clinically-evident infections are included, then those with subclinical infections may be missed, skewing results. This is an example of:
a. Information bias
b. Selection bias
c. Hypothesis testing
d. Generalizability

64. A 28-year-old male with extensive second and third-degree burns develops abdominal discomfort and vomits coffee ground emesis and frank blood. The most likely cause is:
a. A peptic ulcer
b. The erosion of the esophagus from burns
c. Paralytic ileus
d. Stress-related erosive syndrome

65. Beck's triad (increased central venous pressure with distended neck veins, muffled heart sounds, and hypotension) is indicative of which condition?
a. Myocardial infarction
b. Aortic valve prolapse
c. Cardiac tamponade
d. Pulmonary embolism

66. Two months after an ischemic stroke, a patient has difficulty understanding and producing language in speaking, reading, and writing but can understand gestures, pictures, and diagrams. This type of aphasia is:
a. Global
b. Transient
c. Broca's
d. Wernicke's

67. A patient with kidney failure exhibits tachycardia, muscle cramping, hyperreflexia, tetany, nausea, and diarrhea. The most likely cause is:
a. Hypercalcemia

b. Hyperkalemia
c. Hypernatremia
d. Hyperphosphatemia

68. A patient with a recent diagnosis of Parkinson's disease has exhibited positive symptom control from medications but develops mood changes, loss of interest in usual activities, loss of appetite and weight, fatigue, anxiety and insomnia. The most likely cause is:
a. Concern over the condition.
b. Depression.
c. Parkinson's dementia.
d. Inadequate medical control of Parkinson's disease.

69. A patient with pulmonary arterial hypertension most likely has hypertrophy of the:
a. Right atrium.
b. Right ventricle.
c. Left atrium.
d. Left ventricle.

70. A patient with ventricular tachycardia (VT) at 200 bpm and multiple PVCs loses consciousness. Which of the following treatment options is most commonly administered?
a. Antiarrhythmic medications
b. Emergency defibrillation
c. Digoxin
d. Procainamide

71. After cardiac catheterization and removal of the sheath from the femoral artery, a manual compression device is applied and usually inflated to:
a. The patient's current systolic pressure
b. 20 mm Hg above the patient's diastolic pressure
c. 20 mm Hg below the patient's systolic pressure
d. 20 mm Hg above the patient's systolic pressure

72. A patient presents with acute bronchitis with moist productive cough associated with dyspnea, crackling râles, and expiratory high-pitched sibilant wheeze but no fever, and normal white count. The proper treatment includes:

- 139 -

Copyright © Mometrix Media. You have been licensed one copy of this document for personal use only. Any other reproduction or redistribution is strictly prohibited. All rights reserved.

a. Bronchodilators and antibiotics to prevent bacterial infection
b. Antibiotics and a cough suppressant
c. Bronchodilators and a cough suppressant
d. Antibiotics and antihistamines

73. A legal document that specifically designates someone to make decisions regarding medical and end-of-life care for mentally incompetent patients is a(n):
a. Advance Directive
b. Do-Not-Resuscitate Order
c. Durable Power of Attorney
d. General Power of Attorney

74. A 28-year-old diabetic patient has had severe stomach flu rendering him unable to eat solid foods for three days, but has continued to take his regular dose of insulin. He presents with altered consciousness, lethargy, diaphoresis, tremor, tachycardia, and palpitations. Based on his symptoms, his blood glucose level is probably:
a. 100 to 120 mg/dL
b. 81 to 100 mg/dL
c. 70 to 80 mg/dL
d. <70 mg/dL

75. On an electrocardiogram, ischemia is characterized by:
a. Elevation of the ST segment and elevated symmetrical T waves
b. Inverted T wave
c. Development of Q or QS waves
d. Abnormal Q wave or decreased elevation of the R wave without alterations of ST and T waves

76. A patient has severe status asthmaticus and is being evaluated for mechanical ventilation. Which is an absolute indicator of the need for intubation and ventilation?
a. Bradycardia and absent pulse paradoxus
b. Central cyanosis
c. Sharply diminished breath sounds and no audible wheezing
d. Exhaustion/muscle fatigue from exertion of trying to breathe

77. Which heart sound indicates atrial gallop, often associated with left ventricular hypertrophy, hypertension, or aortic stenosis?
a. S1
b. S2
c. S3
d. S4

78. The first sign of Alzheimer's disease is typically:
a. Long-term memory loss
b. Social withdrawal
c. Short-term memory loss
d. Confusion and disorientation

79. A 40-year-old female with chronic asthma is admitted with an acute episode of wheezing and dyspnea. Her medications include a course of oral corticosteroid (prednisone) followed by inhaled corticosteroids. How many days is the patient likely to receive oral corticosteroids?
a. ≤5 days
b. 7 days
c. 10 days
d. 14 days

80. Anticoagulation therapy should be given prior to:
a. Emergency defibrillation
b. Direct current cardioversion
c. Both direct current and chemical cardioversion
d. Chemical cardioversion

81. Atrial-septal defect is characterized by:
a. Shunting of blood returning from the lungs through the left atrium back to the right atrium and pulmonary circulation.
b. Left to right shunt, increased pulmonary hypertension and right-sided heart failure.
c. Right ventricular hypertrophy from increased pressure in the right ventricle and decreased pulmonary blood flow.
d. Left ventricular wall hypertrophy as it increases pressure to overcome valvular resistance.

82. Which of the following is an appropriate action to assess the fifth cranial nerve?

Copyright © Mometrix Media. You have been licensed one copy of this document for personal use only. Any other reproduction or redistribution is strictly prohibited. All rights reserved.

a. Lightly stroke the forehead, cheek, and jaw, have the patient open the mouth, and palpate the muscles for size and strength.
b. Using a penlight, check the eyes for size, shape, reaction to light and accommodation.
c. Have the patient follow a moving finger with his eyes on the vertical plane.
d. Check balance with tandem gait and Romberg's test and hearing with Weber's test and Rinne's test.

83. The best method to evaluate a patient's educational outcomes related to being taught a procedure is to:
a. Ask the patient for feedback
b. Ask the patient to do a demonstration
c. Give the patient an oral test
d. Give the patient a written test

84. A patient has a tracheostomy and requires regular suctioning. What vacuum pressure is appropriate for suctioning a tracheostomy tube?
a. 40 to 60 mm Hg
b. 60 to 80 mm Hg
c. 80 to 100 mm Hg
d. 100 to 120 mm Hg

85. A patient receiving unfractionated heparin therapy develops a sudden drop in platelet count to 45,000 mm³ from a baseline of 120,000 mm³ after 5 days of treatment, suggesting heparin-induced thrombocytopenia. The patient is at risk for:
a. Hemorrhage
b. Thrombosis and vessel occlusion
c. Shock
d. Infection

86. With hypovolemic shock, absolute fluid loss caused by hemorrhage with loss of 30% to 40% of total circulating volume (1500 to 2000 mL) and heart rate >120 with hypotension is classified as:
a. Class I
b. Class II
c. Class III
d. Class IV

87. A patient requires a non-rebreather mask. What action must be completed first?
a. Fit the mask over the nose and mouth
b. Position the elastic strap used to secure the mask
c. Inflate the reservoir to approximately 1 liter with oxygen at 8 to 15 L/min
d. Install the one-way valve

88. The jugular venous pulse can be used to assess:
a. Right atrial function
b. Left atrial function
c. Right ventricular function
d. Left ventricular function

89. A patient receives conscious sedation for a procedure with midazolam and fentanyl. Onset of sedation with midazolam occurs:
a. In 1 to 5 minutes
b. In 6 to 10 minutes
c. In 11 to 15 minutes
d. Immediately

90. When doing research, which of the following sources are NOT valid?
a. Juried medical journal.
b. Popular press report.
c. Professional physician's association.
d. Chief of medical staff.

91. A patient requires a 12-lead electrocardiogram. Where is the V4 precordial lead placed?
a. Right sternal border at the 4th intercostal space
b. Left sternal border at the 4th intercostal space
c. Midway between V4 and V3
d. Left midclavicular line at the 5th intercostal space

Copyright © Mometrix Media. You have been licensed one copy of this document for personal use only. Any other reproduction or redistribution is strictly prohibited. All rights reserved.

92. Electrocardiograph changes characteristic of hypokalemia include:
   a. Peaked T waves with widening and increased amplitude of QRS and prolongation of the QT interval
   b. U wave more than 1 mm high after the T wave, AV block, and flat or inverted T waves
   c. Dysrhythmias with prolonged PR and QT intervals and broad, flat T waves
   d. Nonspecific changes

93. Which of the following diagnoses is characterized by marked elevations of blood pressure that can cause severe organ damage if left untreated?
   a. Aortic aneurysm
   b. Primary hypertension
   c. Secondary hypertension
   d. Hypertensive crisis

94. Which of the following vasodilators primarily dilates coronary arteries and is used to treat angina and supraventricular tachycardia?
   a. Diltiazem (Cardizem®)
   b. Capoten (Captopril®)
   c. Nitroglycerine
   d. Sodium nitroprusside (Nipride®)

95. A newly hired nurse is assisting her team leader, who is preparing to insert an IV catheter. The team leader drops the sterile catheter onto the bed linens and then picks up the contaminated catheter and continues to prepare for insertion. Which of the following responses is the most appropriate for the newly hired nurse?
   a. Wait until the team leader finishes the procedure and ask why she used the contaminated catheter.
   b. Report the team leader's behavior to a supervisor after the catheter is inserted.
   c. Say nothing to anyone, as the linens were clean.
   d. Immediately say: "The catheter was contaminated when it fell. Would you like me to get another setup or stay with the patient while you get it?"

96. Which of the following conditions is associated with uremic syndrome related to end-stage renal disease (ESRD)?
   a. Hypokalemia
   b. Erythrocytopenia
   c. Metabolic alkalosis
   d. Thrombocytosis

97. Which of the following blood abnormalities is a common finding with obstructive sleep apnea?
   a. Increased hematocrit
   b. Decreased hematocrit
   c. Leukopenia
   d. Leukocytosis

98. Which members of the healthcare institution are responsible for identifying quality performance improvement projects?
   a. Administrative staff
   b. Nursing team leaders
   c. Physicians
   d. All staff

99. A patient is recovering from open-heart surgery. Which of the following electrolyte values is outside of the normal range?
   a. Potassium: 3.8 mEq/L
   b. Sodium: 128 mEq/L
   c. Calcium: 9 mg/100 mL
   d. Magnesium: 2 mEq/L

100. In which type of AV block are there more P waves than QRS with no clear relationship between them and an atrial rate 2 to 3 times the pulse rate, with an irregular PR interval?
   a. First degree
   b. Second degree, Mobitz type I
   c. Second degree, Mobitz type II
   d. Third degree

101. Working for the best interests of the patient despite personal values in conflict and assisting patients to have access to appropriate resources comprise:
   a. Moral Agency
   b. Advocacy
   c. Agency
   d. Collaboration

Copyright © Mometrix Media. You have been licensed one copy of this document for personal use only. Any other reproduction or redistribution is strictly prohibited. All rights reserved.

102. A 22 year-old male presents with severe headache, nausea, vomiting, and nuchal rigidity, progressing to confusion, stupor and coma with decerebrate rigidity. This is indicative of:
- a. Subdural hemorrhage
- b. Stroke
- c. Hemorrhage
- d. Hematoma

103. The automatic implantable cardioverter defibrillator (AICD) provides:
- a. (asynchronous) electrical impulses to control pulse rate.
- b. -Chamber sequential electrical impulses.
- c. -Demand (synchronous) electrical impulses when pulse increases to a preset rate.
- d. On-demand electrical impulses when pulse rate decreases to a preset rate.

104. A patient is three hours post–cardiac surgery and is evaluated for renal function. Which of the following findings suggests ineffective renal tissue perfusion?
- a. Specific gravity 1.018
- b. Urinary output: 20 mL/hr
- c. Creatinine (Serum): 0.8 mg/dL
- d. Sodium: 135 mEq/L

105. A patient with a dissecting descending thoracic aortic aneurysm will most likely complain of:
- a. Severe dull pain that builds in intensity in the anterior chest, nausea and vomiting
- b. Severe tearing, knife-like pain that builds in intensity in the anterior chest, nausea and vomiting
- c. , aching posterior pain below the scapula(s), nausea and vomiting
- d. Severe, intense, tearing knife-like posterior pain between the scapulas, nausea and vomiting

106. The nurse is interviewing a patient who is hearing-impaired. Which of the following may be an impediment to communication?
- a. The nurse uses only a normal tone of voice and speaks with short sentences

- b. The nurse provides assistive devices, such as writing materials
- c. The nurse is facing the patient at distance of 8 feet
- d. The nurse uses hand gestures while speaking

107. The best determinant of the effectiveness of teaching is:
- a. Patient's report of compliance
- b. Patient satisfaction based on surveys
- c. Behavior modification
- d. Instructor's knowledge base

108. Which of the following is NOT a characteristic of peripheral arterial insufficiency?
- a. Skin pale and shiny with rubor on dependency and pallor of foot upon elevation
- b. Brownish discoloration (hemosiderin) around ankles and anterior tibial areas
- c. Painful, deep, circular, often necrotic ulcers on toe tips, toe webs, heels, and other pressure areas
- d. Minimal peripheral edema

109. A patient is receiving warfarin along with other treatment for atrial fibrillation. The international normalized ratio (INR) range should be:
- a. 1.5 to 2
- b. 2 to 3
- c. 3 to 4
- d. >4

110. According to Knowles' principles of adult learning, adult learners tend to be:
- a. Unmotivated
- b. Lacking in self-direction
- c. Practical and goal-oriented
- d. Insecure

111. A patient is being considered for thrombolytic therapy with alteplase tissue-type plasminogen activator (t-PA). Which of the following is a contraindication to thrombolytic therapy?
- a. The patient has a 3.5-cm aortic aneurysm

Copyright © Mometrix Media. You have been licensed one copy of this document for personal use only. Any other reproduction or redistribution is strictly prohibited. All rights reserved.

b. The patient is 2 hours post–onset of symptoms
c. The patient's blood pressure has been 180/90 mm Hg, but is controlled by medication
d. The patient hada previous ischemic stroke 6 months ago

112. A 70-year-old female presents with cardiogenic shock secondary to myocardial infarction. Which symptoms are consistent with cardiogenic shock?

a. Hypertension with systolic BP >90 mm Hg, bradycardia <60 bpm with dysrhythmias, chest pain, and tachypnea.
b. Hypotension with systolic BP <90 mm Hg, tachycardia >100 bpm with dysrhythmias, and tachypnea.
c. Hypotension with systolic BP <90 mm Hg, dysrhythmias with varying heart rate, and slow labored respirations.
d. Hypotension with systolic BP <100 mm Hg, bradycardia <60 bpm with regular pulse; and slow, labored respirations.

113. Which of the following medications may be used after cardiac surgery to treat low cardiac output?

a. Nitroprusside
b. Dobutamine
c. Dopamine
d. Isoproterenol

114. A 76 year-old female is being treated for acute heart failure. Testing indicates enlarged ventricles with weak contractions she has developed atrial fibrillation. Which medications will she likely receive?

a. Diuretic, vasodilator, digoxin, and anticoagulant.
b. Diuretic, digoxin, and vasodilator.
c. Diuretic and anticoagulant.
d. Diuretic and vasodilator.

115. A 62 year-old male patient has a regular pulse >100 bpm with P waves before QRS but sometimes preceding the T wave. QRS is of normal shape and duration. PR interval is 0.12 to 0.20 seconds and P: QRS ratio is 1:1. The cardiac diagnosis is:

a. Bradycardia
b. Tachycardia
c. Arrhythmia
d. Atrial contractions

116. Acquired immunodeficiency syndrome (AIDS) is diagnosed when the following criteria are met:

a. HIV infection and AIDS-defining condition, such as cytomegalovirus.
b. HIV infection and CD4 count ≤400 cells/mm$^3$.
c. HIV infection, CD4 count <100 cells/mm$^3$, and AIDS-defining condition.
d. HIV infection, CD4 count <200 cells/mm$^3$, and AIDS-defining condition.

117. Upon physical examination a 23-year-old female complains of chest pain and faintness upon exertion, fatigue, and loss of appetite. She has tachycardia with a weak pulse. Auscultation identifies an ejection click, a brief high-pitched sound occurring immediately after SI. Which of the following cardiac disorders is the most likely diagnosis?

a. Coronary artery disease
b. Mitral valve stenosis
c. Pericarditis
d. Aortic valve stenosis

118. Which of the following rhythm disturbances is most common after cardiac surgery?

a. Ventricular fibrillation
b. Ventricular tachycardia
c. Premature ventricular contractions (PVCs)
d. Atrial fibrillation, flutter, and tachycardia

*Copyright © Mometrix Media. You have been licensed one copy of this document for personal use only. Any other reproduction or redistribution is strictly prohibited. All rights reserved.*

119. A 64 year-old male with chronic heart failure presents with dyspnea, cough, blood-tinged frothy sputum, cyanosis, wheezing, râles, rhonchi, and diaphoresis. He is diagnosed with pulmonary edema, placed on oxygen by mask and given morphine and IV nitrate as well as inhaled aminophylline for bronchospasm. Which of the following diuretics is the most appropriate concomitant treatment option?

a. Furosemide (Lasix ®)
b. Spironolactone (Aldactone ®)
c. Hydrochlorothiazide (Dyazide ®)
d. Eplerenone (Inspra ®)

120. Systemic inflammatory response syndrome (SIRS) is characterized by symptoms that may include:

a. Bradycardia
b. Dysrhythmia
c. Leukocytosis (>12,000 mm³) or leukopenia (<4000 mm³)
d. $PaCO_2$ >32 mm Hg

121. A patient has been receiving heparin for 5 days and develops type I heparin-induced thrombocytopenia and thrombosis syndrome (HITTS) with platelet count of 90,000 mm³. Which of the following actions regarding heparin is most appropriate?

a. Continue heparin, but monitor
b. Stop heparin immediately
c. Reduce dosage of heparin
d. Switch to oral anticoagulants

122. When considering the use of a translator for a patient who does not speak English which of the following considerations is of the highest importance?

a. The translator has training in medical vocabulary for both languages
b. The translator speaks both languages well
c. The translator knows the patient's history
d. The translator is available onsite

123. Which of the following aneurysms would likely require immediate surgical repair?

a. A dissecting 6cm aneurysm in the ascending aorta
b. A 3.5cm saccular abdominal aneurysm

c. A 4cm bulging thoracic aneurysm in the ascending aorta in a patient with Marfan's syndrome
d. A 5cm fusiform abdominal aneurysm

124. A patient with a seizure disorder falls to the floor with a generalized (grand mal) seizure. Which of the following options is the most appropriate nursing action?

a. Position the patient flat on his back and loosen his clothing
b. Open the jaws and insert a padded tongue blade between the teeth
c. Position the patient on one side with the head flexed forward
d. Do not touch the patient until the seizure subsides

125. Angiotensin-converting enzyme (ACE) inhibitors are contraindicated with:

a. Hypertension
b. Diabetes mellitus
c. Heart failure
d. Renal failure.

- 145 -

Copyright © Mometrix Media. You have been licensed one copy of this document for personal use only. Any other reproduction or redistribution is strictly prohibited. All rights reserved.

## Answers and Explanations

1. B: Variant angina (also known as Prinzmetal's angina) results from spasms of the coronary arteries associated with or without atherosclerotic plaques; and is often related to smoking, alcohol, or illicit stimulants. Elevation of ST segments typically occurs with variant angina, which frequently occurs cyclically at the same time each day and often while the person is at rest. Stable angina occurs regularly with activity. Unstable angina occurs when there is a change in the pattern of stable angina. GERD pain may be mistaken for angina.

2. C: Metabolic syndrome (insulin resistance) puts people at risk for the development of diabetes mellitus and cardiovascular disease, and is characterized by abdominal obesity (>35 inches in women and >40 inches in men), increased triglycerides (≥150), decreased HDL level (<40 mm Hg in men and <50 mm Hg in women), elevation of blood pressure (≥130/≥85 mm Hg), and increased fasting glucose (≥110 mg/dL). Other indicators include elevation of C-reactive protein (evidence of a proinflammatory state) and high levels of fibrinogen (evidence of a prothrombotic state).

3. C: The total nutrient admixture should be discarded if there is "cracking" of the lipid emulsion and the oil separates into a layer. With TNA, all the components of parenteral nutrition and lipids are admixed together in one container to create a 3-in-1 formula. Components of parenteral nutrition generally include proteins, carbohydrates, fats, electrolytes, vitamins, sterile water, and trace vitamins. While most postoperative patients need 1500 calories per day to prevent protein breakdown, those with fever, burns, major surgery, trauma, or hypermetabolic disease may need up to 10,000 more calories daily.

4. B: The nurse should give morphine, as 8 on a 1 to 10 scale is representative of severe pain, not uncommon in the first 24 hours after surgery.

Patients have a right to pain control, and the nurse should trust that the pain is what the patient says it is. Patients may show very different behavior when they are in pain. Some may cry and moan with minor pain, and others may exhibit little difference in behavior when truly suffering. Thus, judging pain by behavior can lead to the wrong conclusions. Questioning family members is not appropriate.

5. D: Q-wave myocardial infarction is characterized by complete coronary occlusion in 80% to 90% of patients. Abnormal Q waves (wider and deeper) are especially common in the morning. Infarction is usually prolonged, resulting in transmural necrosis. Peak CK levels occur in approximately 27 hours. Non-Q-wave myocardial infarction is characterized by ST changes with ST depression. Infarct is typically non-transmural and small with coronary occlusion in only 20% to 30% of patients. Peak CK levels occur in approximately 12 to 13 hours.

6. C: The nurse who delegates remains accountable for patient outcomes and for supervision of the person to whom the task was delegated. The scope of nursing includes delegation of tasks to unlicensed assistive personnel, providing those personnel have adequate training and knowledge. Delegation can be used to manage the workload and to provide adequate and safe care. Delegation should be done in a manner that reduces liability by providing adequate communication.

7. B: Acute lung injury results in severely compromised lungs with crackling râles and wheezing, decreased pulmonary compliance, and cyanosis, so oxygen therapy is provided to maintain oxygen saturation >90%. Oxygen should be administered at 100% because of the mismatch between ventilation (V) and perfusion (Q), which can result in hypoxia upon change in positioning. Endotracheal intubation may be needed if oxygen saturation falls or carbon dioxide levels rise.

8. C: The normal BUN/creatinine ratio is 10:1. Normal serum creatinine is 0.6 to 1.2 mg/dL)

Copyright © Mometrix Media. You have been licensed one copy of this document for personal use only. Any other reproduction or redistribution is strictly prohibited. All rights reserved.

and increases with impaired renal function, urinary tract obstruction, and nephritis. Levels should remain stable with normal functioning. Normal blood urea nitrogen (BUN) is 7 to 8 mg/dL for patients younger than age 60, and 8 to 20 mg/dL for patients 60 years of age and older. BUN increases with hypovolemia. The ratio remains normal with intrinsic kidney disease but both the BUN and creatinine levels are increased.

9. A: An MI causes damage to the myocardium in stages beginning when ischemia develops, creating a zone of ischemia with viable cells. Cellular injury then occurs to those cells surrounding the infarcted area in the zone of injury. Infarction with necrosis of tissue comprises the zone of infarction, where cells are destroyed and eventually replaced with scar tissue. People may exhibit either hypertension or hypotension during an MI.

10. A: The most common initial treatment of acute pulmonary edema is oxygen to relieve dyspnea, nitroglycerine to reduce preload, loop diuretics, usually furosemide, to promote diuresis and venodilation, and morphine to reduce associated anxiety (although some doctors avoid morphine because of side effects). ACE inhibitors are also sometimes used to reduce afterload, but thiazide diuretics are not used to treat acute pulmonary edema. Calcium channel blockers may induce acute pulmonary edema if used with tocolytics.

11. B: Polyvinyl (hydrophilic) non-adherent porous foam is used for all wounds except deep wound with moderate granulation, deep pressure ulcers, and flaps. Polyurethane (hydrophobic, repelling moisture) is used for all wounds except those that are painful, have tunneling or sinus tracts, deep trauma wounds, and wounds needing controlled growth of granulation. The foam is cut to fit and cover the wound and is secured with foam-occlusive transparent film. An opening is cut to accommodate the drainage tube, which is attached to a suction canister, creating a closed system with pressure set to a range of 75 to 125.

12. A: The 60-year-old male is most likely to experience classic signs of a myocardial infarction, as they are most common in males. Females and those under 55 often present with atypical symptoms. Diabetic patients may have reduced sensation of pain due to neuropathy and may complain primarily of weakness. Elderly patients may also have neuropathic changes that reduce sensation of pain.

13. D: The Health Insurance Portability and Accountability Act (HIPAA) addresses the rights of the individual related to privacy of health information. The nurse must not release any information or documentation about a patient's condition or treatment without consent, as the individual has the right to determine who has access to personal information, which is considered protected health information (PHI), including health history, condition, treatments in any form, and any documentation. Personal information can be shared with spouse, legal guardians, and those with durable power of attorney.

14. B: Hepatitis A is transmitted by the oral-fecal route, often from contamination on the hands or through sexual contact. Outbreaks have been traced to restaurants and kitchens in large facilities. Hepatitis B is transmitted through blood and body fluids, such as through sexual contact or sharing needles. Hepatitis C is transmitted directly through blood or items, such as shared needles contaminated with blood, and sexual contact. Fulminant hepatitis is an acute liver infection triggered by hepatitis or other viruses, toxins (carbon tetrachloride), Wilson's disease, and drugs, most commonly Tylenol ® (acetaminophen).

15. D: The patient is experiencing the stage of bargaining during which patient/family may change doctors, trying to change the outcome. People grieve individually and may not go through all stages, but most go through at least 2 stages. Kübler-Ross's 5 stages of grief include:
1. Denial: Disbelieving, confused, stunned, detached, repeating questions.

*Copyright © Mometrix Media. You have been licensed one copy of this document for personal use only. Any other reproduction or redistribution is strictly prohibited. All rights reserved.*

2. Anger: Directed inward (self-blame) or outward.
3. Bargaining: If- then thinking. (If I go to church, then I will heal.) Trying to find a different outcome.
4. Depression: Sad, withdrawn, tearful, crying but beginning to accept loss.
5. Acceptance: Resolution and acceptance.

16. A: The most likely diagnosis is foreign-body aspiration. Patients with advanced Parkinson's disease often have dysphagia and are prone to aspiration. Foreign body aspiration can cause obstruction of the pharynx, larynx, or trachea, leading to acute dyspnea or asphyxiation, and the object may be drawn distally into the bronchial tree. With adults, most foreign bodies migrate more readily down the right bronchus. Objects in the bronchus cause cough, dyspnea, and wheezing.

17. D: Troponin (protein in the myocardium) and its isomers (C, I, and T) regulate contractions, and levels increases as with CK-MB after an MI, but levels remain elevated for up to three weeks. An ECG is most helpful if taken immediately after an MI so heart changes over time can be monitored. Myoglobin levels increase in 1 to 3 hours after an MI and peak within 12 hours. CK-MB levels increase within a few hours and peak at about 24-27 hours (earlier with thrombolytic therapy or PTCA) for Q-wave MI and 12-13 hours for non–Q-wave MI.

18. B: These symptoms are typical of metabolic alkalosis: Elevated serum pH, $PCO_2$ relatively normal (if compensated) or increased (if uncompensated), and urine pH >6 (if compensated). The patient is dizzy, confused, and is exhibiting tremors, seizures, tingling, tachycardia, and arrhythmias. Metabolic alkalosis occurs with decreased strong acid or increased base, with compensatory $CO_2$ retention by the lungs associated with hypoventilation. Metabolic alkalosis is usually caused by excessive vomiting, gastric suctioning, diuretics, potassium deficit, excessive mineralocorticoids, and/or excessive $NaHCO_3$ intake.

19. A: The correct action is to reduce the osmolality of the solution to prevent dumping syndrome. A concentrated solution with high osmolality can draw fluid into the stomach and intestines from the surrounding tissues and the blood, causing abdominal discomfort and fullness, nausea, and diarrhea, leading to dehydration and a drop in blood pressure and increased heart rate. Patients who are weak are more prone to dumping syndrome. Reducing the osmolality and gradually increasing it allows the body to adjust and relieves symptoms.

20. B: Endocarditis is characterized by Janeway lesions (painless areas of hemorrhage on the palms of the hands and soles of the feet), splinter hemorrhages on the nails, petechiae on the oral mucosa, and Roth's spots (hemorrhagic lesions on the retina caused by emboli on nerve fibers). Other symptoms include slow onset with low-grade or intermittent fever, anorexia, weight loss, fatigue, anemia, splenomegaly, hepatomegaly, cyanosis and clubbing of fingers, CHF, heart murmur, and embolism to other body organs (brain, liver, bones).

21. D: Severe dehydration is fluid loss >15% and occurs when total body water decreases but sodium does not. It is characterized by marked hypotension and anuria as well as symptoms associated with lesser dehydration. Mild dehydration (5% loss) is characterized by dizziness, lethargy, reduced skin turgor, dry mucous membranes, and orthostatic hypotension. Moderate dehydration (10% loss) is characterized by confusion, resting hypotension, tachycardia, and oliguria/anuria. Dehydration may result from inadequate fluids, excess water loss, NG suctioning, drugs, diarrhea, vomiting, and fever.

22. C: Neurogenic shock is often characterized by bradycardia, hypotension, and warm dry skin related to lack of vascular tone that results in hypothermia from loss of cutaneous heat. Neurogenic shock can occur when spinal cord injury, neurological disease, drugs, or anesthesia impairs the autonomic nervous system that controls the cardiovascular system.

Copyright © Mometrix Media. You have been licensed one copy of this document for personal use only. Any other reproduction or redistribution is strictly prohibited. All rights reserved.

23. D: Open-ended questions, such as "Is there anything you'd like to discuss?" encourage patients to express feelings. Nurses should avoid meaningless clichés, such as "Don't worry. Everything will be fine," as this may not be true, and should avoid providing direct advice with "You should…" or "The best thing to do is…," but should provide facts and encourage patients to make decisions. "Why are you upset?" questions behavior that may not directly relate to care and requires analysis of feelings.

24. A: Patients with chronic ventilatory failure cannot compensate for hypercapnia and the pH falls, resulting in respiratory acidosis. Symptoms include increasing dyspnea with tachypnea, gasping respirations, and use of accessory muscles. Patients may become confused as hypercapnia causes increased intracranial pressure. If pH is <7.2, cardiac arrhythmias, hyperkalemia, and hypotension can occur as pulmonary arteries constrict and the peripheral vascular system dilates. ABGs are consistent with respiratory acidosis ($PCO_2$ >50 and pH<7.35).

25. D: The best time to initiate conflict resolution is when conflict first emerges, but before open conflict and hardening of positions. Steps include:

- Allowing both parties to present their sides without bias.
- Encouraging operation through negotiation and compromise.
- Maintaining focus and avoiding arguments.
- Evaluating the need for renegotiation, formal resolution process, or third party.
- Utilizing humor and empathy to diffuse tension.
- Summarizing and outlining key arguments.
- Avoiding forcing resolution if possible.

26. A: These symptoms are typical of a stroke in the right hemisphere. A left hemispheric stroke results in right-sided paresis and visual field defect. Depression and cautious behavior is common. Patients have math and language difficulties that can include aphasia and difficulty with reading and writing. Patients may have short-term memory loss and difficulty learning new material. Brain stem stroke impairs cardiac and respiratory function and often results in death. Cerebellum stroke results in ataxia, nausea, vomiting, headache, and dizziness or vertigo.

27. C: Pericarditis is treated with anti-inflammatory drugs, such as aspirin or ibuprofen, activity restriction, and sometimes corticosteroids. Surgical intervention may include pericardiocentesis, which is removing fluid from the pericardial sac in order to relieve increasing pressure and to diagnose the causative agent. In some cases, a small opening may be made into the pericardium to allow continuous drainage of exudate into the chest cavity. In severe cases, the outer layer of the pericardium may be removed if it is preventing functioning of the ventricles.

28. D: The "5 rights of delegation" include:
1. Task: The nurse determines as appropriate task to delegate for a specific patient.
2. Circumstance: The nurse has considered all relevant information to determine the appropriateness of delegation.
3. Person: The nurse chooses the right person based on education and skills to perform the task.
4. Direction: The nurse provides a clear description of the task, purpose, limits, and expected outcomes.
5. Supervision: The nurse can supervise, intervene as needed, and evaluate performance.

29. C: This patient is exhibiting signs of ketoacidosis, so initial treatment will include insulin therapy per continuous infusion and fluid (non-glucose) and electrolyte therapy. Typical

*Copyright © Mometrix Media. You have been licensed one copy of this document for personal use only. Any other reproduction or redistribution is strictly prohibited. All rights reserved.*

symptoms include Kussmaul respirations (hyperventilation with "ketone breath" to eliminate carbon dioxide), fluid imbalance with loss of potassium and other electrolytes from cellular death resulting in dehydration from diuresis with excess thirst, cardiac arrhythmias from potassium decline, and hyperglycemia (blood glucose 300 to 800 mg/dL).

30. A: PCR of a biopsy specimen yields the most accurate diagnostic results for myocarditis. An echocardiogram may indicate cardiomegaly and defects in functioning. ECG changes may be non-specific. Cardiac catheterization and cardiac biopsy will yield confirmation in 65% of cases, but not all of the heart muscle may be affected, so a negative finding does not rule out myocarditis. Other tests include chest radiograph to indicate cardiomegaly or pulmonary edema and viral cultures of the nasopharynx and rectum to identify organism. Viral titres may increase with disease progression.

31. D: Theophylline is usually not initiated with acute exacerbations unless there is no response to short-and/or long-acting bronchodilators or corticosteroids. Short-acting bronchodilators (albuterol) treat bronchospasm and airway obstruction, but should be discontinued if ineffective. Long-acting bronchodilators (eg. formoterol and salmeterol) are often more effective. Other treatments include inhaled and oral corticosteroids, supplemental oxygen, antibiotics if change in character of sputum, and chest physiotherapy.

32. D: The leader who wants everyone to follow the organization's rules exactly is bureaucratic. Autocratic leaders make decisions independently and enforce rules while charismatic leaders rely on personal charm to influence and persuade. Consultative leaders present a decision and welcome input but rarely change decisions while participatory leaders present potential decisions but make final decisions based on input. Democratic leaders present the problem and ask teams to arrive at a solution. Laissez-faire leaders exert little control and allow staff to make decisions with little interference.

33. A: Balloon valvuloplasty of the aortic valve is probably not indicated because aortic valves are tricuspid (3 leaflets) and repair is not typically possible, so defective valves must be replaced with mechanical (metal, plastic or pyrolytic carbon) or biological (porcine or bovine) xenografts. The Ross procedure uses the patient's pulmonary artery with the pulmonary valve to replace the aortic valve and part of the aorta and then uses a donor graft to replace the pulmonary artery. An aortic homograft uses a donor's aorta with the aortic valve attached.

34. C: Hemoglobin A1C of 5.5% most indicates dietary compliance. Hemoglobin AIC comprises hemoglobin A with a glucose molecule because hemoglobin holds onto excess blood glucose, so it shows the average blood glucose levels over a three month period and is used primarily to monitor long-term diabetic therapy: Normal value: <6% and elevation >7%. Fasting blood sugar (FBS) results can vary widely but show current serum level, so a person who stays on a diet for a few days and fasts may show a near-normal FBS for a short period even though the patient is frequently non-compliant. Normal FBS: 70 to 99 mg/dL.

35. B: The patient most likely has developed paralytic ileus (paralysis of the bowel), which can result from infection (such as pancreatitis), narcotics, excessive manipulation during surgery, and prolonged anesthesia. Symptoms of bowel obstruction are similar but often more

Copyright © Mometrix Media. You have been licensed one copy of this document for personal use only. Any other reproduction or redistribution is strictly prohibited. All rights reserved.

severe with abdominal rigidity, shock, respiratory distress, and sepsis. Bowel infarction causes acute abdomen and shock. Short gut (bowel) syndrome results from a malabsorptive condition after removal of part of the small intestine.

36. D: A thoracentesis may be done with the patient lying on the opposite side with the head of the bed elevated 30° to 45° so that fluid remains at the base of the lung. The patient should avoid coughing or moving during the procedure. Placement is determined by chest x-ray or ultrasound. A local anesthetic is administered and a needle (with a 20-mL syringe and 3-way stopcock with tubing and a receptacle) is advanced intercostally into the pleural space to collect fluid. A pressure dressing is applied when needle is removed. A chest x-ray checks for pneumothorax.

37. B: Under the ANA Nursing Code of Ethics, autonomy and self-determination are viewed within the broad context of diverse cultures. The idea of individualism is less important in some cultures, so the nurse must respect and appreciate the patient's right to be guided by her family. Trying to convince the patient to assert herself may just lead to emotional conflict. This is not an appropriate concern for the ethics committee, as the woman is not being forced to comply with family decisions but chooses to do so.

38. B: Caffeinated foods (tea, coffee, and hot chocolate) may increase the effects of warfarin. Alcohol intake should be limited to no more than 3 drinks daily. A daily multivitamin should not affect warfarin, but some herbal medications can affect clotting time. Milk products should not affect warfarin, but foods that are high in vitamin K may affect the medication, and should be limited and eaten in consistent amounts. These include broccoli, green leafy vegetables (kale, turnip greens, and beet greens), cauliflower, and legumes as well as soybean and canola oils.

39. C: Laboratory abnormalities with DIC include prolonged prothrombin and partial prothrombin times and decreased platelet count and fibrinogen with fragmented RBCs. Treatment includes identifying underlying cause, blood replacement products, and anticoagulation therapy to increase clotting time, cryoprecipitate to increase fibrinogen levels, and coagulation inhibitors and coagulation factors.

40. A: While all of these conditions may cause similar symptoms, the sudden onset and fluctuating nature indicate delirium. Delirium occurs in approximately 80% of terminally ill patients and may result from drugs, such as anticholinergics and hypnotics. Delirium may also occur with numerous other conditions, including infection, hypoxia, trauma, dementia, depression, hearing and/or vision loss, surgery, alcoholism, untreated pain, fluid/electrolyte balance, and malnutrition.

41. B: The leader should prepare a detailed agenda for topics of discussion before the meeting. Adding topics during the meeting just takes time and adds to the confusion. Asking for topics at the beginning of the meeting is time-consuming and can devolve into conflict and discussions that are non-productive. Free discussions may lead to topics of discussion but little time is left for dealing with issues.

42. A: Hyperkalemia often occurs with renal disease and is characterized by ventricular arrhythmia, weakness with ascending paralysis and hyperreflexia, diarrhea, and confusion. Hypokalemia is characterized by weakness, lethargy, nausea and vomiting, paresthesias, dysrhythmias (PVCs, flattened T waves), muscle cramps with hyporeflexia, hypotension, and tetany. Hypocalcemia is characterized by tetany, tingling, seizures, altered mental status, and ventricular tachycardia. Hypercalcemia is characterized by increasing muscle weakness with hypotonicity, constipation, anorexia, nausea and vomiting, and bradycardia.

43. D: This PCTA patient is probably experiencing a retroperitoneal arterial bleed into the flank area, requiring cessation of anticoagulants and preparations for IV fluids and/or blood. Bleeding or hematoma at the

Copyright © Mometrix Media. You have been licensed one copy of this document for personal use only. Any other reproduction or redistribution is strictly prohibited. All rights reserved.

sheath site is treated by laying the patient flat and applying pressure to the sheath site. Ultrasound-guided compression and surgery is indicated if pulsatile mass or bruit occurs near insertion site, indicating pseudoaneurysm or arteriovenous fistula. Anticoagulation therapy is indicated for decreased circulation in extremity related to thrombus or embolus.

44. C: An autologous blood patch (15 to 20 mL) is injected epidurally near the subarachnoid puncture site to plug the puncture hole in the dura. Postdural puncture headache (frontal and/or occipital) results from loss of cerebrospinal fluid through the puncture hole, resulting in posterior displacement of the brainand stress on supporting structures. Headache onset is usually 12 to 48 hours after puncture but may be delayed for weeks or months. Conservative treatment includes bed rest, fluid, and caffeine.

45. A: These are signs of cocaine use, both inhaled (nasal irritation and nosebleeds) and smoked (lip burns, cough). Constricted pupils, headaches, and abdominal pain are common. Most abused drugs have similar symptoms. However, heroin users would have needle tracks and would not have nasal irritation. Marijuana users may exhibit tachycardia and cough from lung irritation (similar to tobacco smokers), but usually do not develop nasal irritation or nose bleeds. Methadone abuse can cause constricted pupils and abdominal pain, but does not cause nasal symptoms.

46. D: With the 3-chamber water seal (wet suction) system, the first chamber is for collection, and sterile water is instilled into the middle water seal and third wet suction chambers. With a 3-chamber dry water seal system, sterile fluid is instilled to the 2cm level in the water seal chamber only. The 2-chambered dry suction system requires no fluid instillation.

47. C: ReoPro ® (abciximab) is contraindicated with recent history of oral anticoagulation (warfarin), recent bleeding or stroke within the previous 2 years, or platelet count <100,000 mm. ³. ReoPro ®is used to prevent cardiac ischemia for those undergoing percutaneous cardiac intervention, such as for angina. ReoPro ® inhibits the aggregation of platelets and is used with aspirin and/or weight-adjusted, low-dose heparin as it potentiates the action of anticoagulants. However, its use with non–weight adjusted longer-acting heparin can cause thrombocytopenia with increased risk of hemorrhage.

48. B: The learner outcome for teaching a patient about insulin reaction should relate directly to that goal List and describe the symptoms of insulin reaction. While all of the other things (different types of insulin, foods high in carbohydrates, and the difference between type 1 diabetes and type 2 diabetes) are important, they don't relate to the topic and should not be the learner outcome for this activity. In some cases, one class or session may cover multiple topics with multiple outcomes, but a patient may be overwhelmed by too much information.

49. D: Disorientation, agitation, hallucinations, and paranoia are indications of postcardiotomy delirium. These symptoms usually appear between 3 and 7 days after surgery, persisting for days or weeks. Neurological status should be evaluated carefully after surgery, especially in the first 48 to 72 hours when subtle changes may become evident. Mild sedation or haloperidol may relieve symptoms.

50. A: Oxygen concentration with nasal cannula ranges from approximately 24% to 44% because it is not an airtight system; some ambient air is breathed in as well. While a nasal cannula can be used to deliver supplemental oxygen, it is only useful for flow rates ≤6 L/min as higher rates are drying of the nasal passages.

51. A: A holistic view of relationships within the organization facilitates problem-solving along with an understanding of how structures, patterns, and events affect outcomes. Those who identify with role rather than purpose may have difficulty understanding the needs of others.

Copyright © Mometrix Media. You have been licensed one copy of this document for personal use only. Any other reproduction or redistribution is strictly prohibited. All rights reserved.

Those who rely too much on past experience may be resistant to change, and a feeling of victimization makes people feel that the organization or leadership is to blame for their own personal shortcomings, and they feel there is nothing they can do to make changes.

52. C: Oxygen saturation should be maintained at >95% although some patients with chronic respiratory disorders, such as COPD may have lower $SPO_2$. Results may be compromised by impaired circulation, excessive light, poor positioning, and nail polish. If $SPO_2$ falls, the oximeter should be repositioned, as incorrect positioning is a common cause of inaccurate readings. Oximetry is often used post surgically and when patients are on mechanical ventilation.

53. D: A small pneumothorax may resolve or stabilize, so the patient should receive oxygen and be observed for 3 to 6 hours. If there is no increase in size on a repeat x-ray, the patient may be discharged but asked to return for another x-ray in 24 to 48 hours. Chest-tube thoracostomy with underwater seal drainage is the most common treatment for all types of pneumothoraces. A tension pneumothorax requires immediate needle decompression followed by chest-tube thoracostomy.

54. A: The heart rate is controlled by the autonomic nervous system, and in a normal heart a decrease in heart rate is usually compensated for by an increase in stroke volume. However, with cardiomyopathy, this may not occur, and bradycardia may cause a decline in cardiac output. Normal cardiac output is about 5 L/min at rest for an adult although this may multiply 3 or 4 times with exercise and stress, with resultant changes in the heart rate and stroke volume.

55. C: Kinesthetic learners learn best by handling, doing, practicing and should be allowed to handle supplies/equipment with minimal directions. They benefit from demonstrating their understanding by doing the procedure. Visual learners learn best by seeing and reading and benefit from written directions, videos, diagrams, pictures, and demonstrations, whereas auditory learners learn best by listening and talking, so procedures should be explained during demonstrations. Auditory learners benefit from audiotapes and extra time for questions.

56. C: Hemorrhage of esophageal varices occurs in approximately one-third of those with portal hypertension and is the most common cause of death with cirrhosis. As the portal vein becomes obstructed increased pressure develops in vessels, especially in the lower esophagus and stomach, causing collateral vessels and varicosities to form. These collateral vessels are fragile and rupture easily. Jaundice, blockage of the bile duct and abdominal distention (ascites) occur with hepatic failure and are generally present prior to the development of portal hypertension.

57. B: Preload may decrease as a result of dehydration, diuresis, or vasodilation. Preload may increase as a result of increased venous return, controlling fluid loss, transfusions, or IV fluids. Preload refers to the amount of elasticity in the myocardium at the end of diastole when the ventricles are filled to their maximum volume and the stretch on the muscle fibers is the greatest. The preload value is based on the volume in the ventricles. The amount of preload (stretch) affects stroke volume because as stretch increases, the resultant contraction also increases (Frank-Starling Law).

58. A: Acute renal failure resulting from prerenal disorders, such as sepsis MI, HF, anaphylaxis, and hemorrhage, is caused by hypoperfusion and decreased glomerular filtration rate. Intrarenal disorders, such as burns and crush trauma, release myoglobin and hemoglobin from tissues, causing toxicity and/or ischemia. Transfusion reactions result in hemolysis with precipitates in the tubules. Some medications, such as NSAIDs and ACE inhibitors may interfere with kidney function and cause hypoperfusion and ischemia. Postrenal disorders involve distal obstruction that increases pressure in tubules and decreases GFR.

*Copyright © Mometrix Media. You have been licensed one copy of this document for personal use only. Any other reproduction or redistribution is strictly prohibited. All rights reserved.*

59. C: This patient is exhibiting signs of pulmonary embolism. While clinical manifestations vary according to the size of the embolus and area of occlusion, common symptoms include dyspnea with tachypnea, cough (sometimes with hemoptysis), râles, and chest pain. Other signs include hiccoughs, tachycardia, hemodynamic instability, anxiety, restlessness and fever. ABG analysis shows hypoxemia ($\downarrow$PaO$_2$), hypocarbia ($\downarrow$PaCO$_2$) and respiratory alkalosis ($\uparrow$pH). D-dimer shows elevation (>500 ng/mL).

60. B: Two sets of bioimpedance electrodes are placed bilaterally at the base of the neck and then two sets on each side of the chest. ECG leads are placed where they consistently monitor the QRS signal, and they may need to be moved to achieve this. Chest electrodes measure changes in electrical output associated with the volume of blood through the aorta and its velocity. The monitor converts the signals to waveforms. The heart rate is shown on an ECG monitor. The equipment calculates the cardiac output based on the heart rate and fluid volume.

61. A: The nurse should attend to the spiritual needs of the patient by calling a priest even though the hour is not convenient. A Protestant chaplain cannot perform specific rituals that are important to Catholics, and the patient may not survive or be able to receive communion if the call is delayed. Catholic rituals include:
- Sacrament of the Anointing of the Sick: This replaces the last rites (Extreme Unction) and is a bedside blessing.
- *Viaticum*: This is essentially the "last" Holy Communion and is called the "food for the journey."

62. A: The nurse should call the mental health crisis team. Crisis teams are comprised of mental health professionals. The teams are typically available to non-psychiatric units in order to evaluate the mental status of a patient. In this case, the patient is most likely experiencing an exacerbation of her bipolar disease as a result of the stress related to surgery, and could

irreparably damage her surgical repair, so the crisis team will determine whether the patient is a danger to herself or others and whether she should remain hospitalized for treatment.

63. B: Selection bias occurs when the method of selecting subjects results in a cohort that is not representative of the target population because of inherent error in design. Information bias occurs when there are errors in classification, so an estimate of association is incorrect. A hypothesis should be generated about the probable cause based on the information available in laboratory and medical records, epidemiologic study, literature review, and expert opinion. Hypothesis testing includes data analysis, laboratory findings, and outcomes of testing. Generalizability is when results of research are true for similar populations.

64. D: Stress-related erosive syndrome (SRES), or stress ulcers, occur most frequently in those who are critically ill, such as those with severe or multi-organ trauma, mechanical ventilation, sepsis, severe burns, and head injury with increased intracranial pressure. Stress induces changes in the gastric mucosal lining and decreased perfusion of the mucosa, causing ischemia. SRES involves hemorrhage in ≥30% of patients with mortality rates of 30% to 80%. The lesions tend to be diffuse, so they are more difficult to treat than peptic ulcers. Symptoms include coffee ground emesis, hematemesis, and abdominal discomfort.

65. C: Beck's triad (increased central venous pressure with distended neck veins, muffled heart sounds, and hypotension) is commonly found with cardiac tamponade. Other symptoms may include a feeling of pressure or pain in the chest as well as dyspnea, and pulsus paradoxus >10 mm Hg (systolic blood pressure heard during exhalation but not during inhalation). Cardiac tamponade occurs with pericardial effusion in which fluid accumulates in the pericardial sac causing pressure against the heart. It may be a complication of trauma, pericarditis, cardiac surgery, or heart failure.

*Copyright © Mometrix Media. You have been licensed one copy of this document for personal use only. Any other reproduction or redistribution is strictly prohibited. All rights reserved.*

66. A: Aphasia is the loss of ability to use and/or understand written or spoken word because of damage to speech centers in the brain. Global aphasia is characterized by difficulty understanding and producing language but patients may understand gestures, pictures, and diagrams. Transient aphasia is short lasting, and often related to transient ischemic episodes. Broca's aphasia is characterized by the ability to understand, but difficulty producing language. Wernicke's aphasia is characterized by difficulty understanding language but ability to understand gestures and produce language.

67. D: Hyperphosphatemia occurs with renal failure as well as hypoparathyroidism, excessive intake, neoplastic diseases, diabetic ketoacidosis, muscle necrosis, and chemotherapy and is associated with hypocalcemia. Symptoms of hyperphosphatemia include tachycardia, muscle cramping, hyperreflexia, tetany, nausea and diarrhea. Treatment includes identifying and treating underlying cause, correcting hypocalcemia, and providing antacids and dialysis.

68. B: The most likely cause is depression caused by medications used to treat Parkinson's disease. Other drugs that can precipitate depression include estrogen, corticosteroids, cimetidine, hydralazine, propanolol, digitalis, and indomethacin. Because the onset develops shortly after beginning therapy, the medication is more likely to blame than concern over condition. Parkinson's dementia usually develops later, and the patient's Parkinson's symptoms are well controlled by the medication.

69. B: Pulmonary arterial hypertension (PAH) may result in right ventricular hypertrophy. Typically the pulmonary vasculature adjusts easily to accommodate blood volume from the right ventricle. If there is increased blood flow, the low resistance causes vasodilation and vice versa. However, sometimes the pulmonary vascular bed is damaged or obstructed, and this can impair the ability to handle changing volumes of blood. In that case, an increase in flow will increase the pulmonary arterial pressure, increasing pulmonary vascular resistance (PVR). This in turn, increases pressure on the right ventricle (RV) with increased RV workload, and eventual RV hypertrophy with displacement of the intraventricular septum and tricuspid regurgitation. Over time, this leads to right-sided heart failure and death.

70. B: Emergency defibrillation is typically performed with VT and unconsciousness. Ventricular tachycardia is associated with ≥3 PVCs in a row and a ventricular rate of 100 to 200 bpm. The rapid rate of contractions makes VT dangerous as the ineffective beats may render the person unconscious with no palpable pulse. A detectable rate is typically regular and the QRS complex is ≥ 0.12 second and (often) abnormally shaped. The P wave may be undetectable with an irregular PR interval if the P wave is present. The P: QRS ratio is difficult to ascertain if the P wave is missing.

71. D: After cardiac catheterization and removal of the sheath, pressure must be applied for 5 to 10 minutes to prevent bleeding and hematoma formation. A manual compression device is applied by a belt around the hips with a pad over the insertion site and then inflated to 20 mm Hg above the patient's systolic pressure in order to promote hemostasis. Digital compression may also be used. Sometimes lidocaine is administered at the site to relieve discomfort, but this may result in a vasovagal response, so atropine (0.6-1.0 mg IV) should be available.

72. C: The best treatment for bronchitis includes bronchodilators and cough suppressant. Because most cases of acute bronchitis are caused by viruses and are self-limiting in 2 to 3 weeks, antibiotics should be avoided unless signs of infection, such as prolonged fever, elevated WBC, or change in character of sputum, occur. Antihistamines may be used for those with allergic triggers. In adults, the most common viral triggers are influenza virus, adenovirus, and respiratory syncytial virus (RSV).

Copyright © Mometrix Media. You have been licensed one copy of this document for personal use only. Any other reproduction or redistribution is strictly prohibited. All rights reserved.

73. C: The legal document that designates someone to make decisions regarding medical and end-of-life care if a patient is mentally incompetent is a Durable Power of Attorney. This is a type of Advance Directive, which can include living wills or specific requests of the patient regarding treatment. A Do-Not-Resuscitate Order indicates that the patient does not want resuscitative treatment for terminal illness or condition. A General Power of Attorney allows a designated person to make decisions for a person over broader areas, including financial.

74. D: This patient exhibits signs of hypoglycemia. Symptoms are usually evident when blood glucose falls below 70 mg/dL. Hypoglycemia almost always results from treatment for diabetes mellitus, such as the use of insulin. In this case, hypoglycemia relates to too much medication (insulin or oral medications) and inadequate nutritional intake. Excessive exercise, illness, and infections that burn glucose stores can also result in hypoglycemia. Because the brain requires glucose to function, an inadequate supply of glucose can affect the central nervous system.

75. B: Ischemia is characterized by inverted T-waves. As the cardiac muscle is damaged, the ST segment is elevated with elevated symmetrical T-waves. With a Q-wave myocardial infarction, Q or QS-waves develop as repolarization is altered or absent. Changes in the Q-wave are often permanent, so an old MI is evidenced by abnormal Q-wave or decreased elevation of the R-wave without alterations of ST and T-waves. Non–Q-wave myocardial infarction does not cause Q-wave changes.

76. A: Bradycardia and absence of pulsus paradoxus are absolute indicators of the need for intubation and mechanical ventilation with status asthmaticus because these indicate imminent respiratory arrest. Additional absolute indicators include marked depression, cardiac and/or pulmonary arrest and severe hypoxia and/or apnea. Other symptoms are evaluated on an individual basis and include central cyanosis, sharply diminished breath sounds, exhaustion, deteriorating mental status, dysphonia, $PaO_2$ <70 mm Hg on 100% $O_2$, pulse paradoxus >20-40 mm Hg, ↑ hypercapnia, metabolic/respiratory acidosis, and pH <7.20.

77. D: S4 is an extra beat (atrial gallop) occurring just prior to S1, producing a triple "Tennessee" rhythm. It is often associated with left ventricular hypertrophy, hypertension, or aortic stenosis. S1 and S2 are normal heart sounds. S1 indicates the onset of systole with closure of both the tricuspid and mitral valves. S2 is the end of systole and indicates closure of the pulmonary and aortic valves. S3 is an extra beat producing a triple rhythm ("Kentucky") and indicates decreased ventricular compliance, often related to left ventricular failure and mitral regurgitation.

78. C: The first sign of Alzheimer's disease is typically short-term memory loss with forgetting of words and misplacement of items. Social withdrawal occurs later with some loss of long-term memory. As the brain continues to atrophy with shrinkage in the cerebral cortex and hippocampus, patients become increasingly confused and disoriented, often forgetting their address and telephone number, and dressing inappropriately, as well as forgetting to eat. This is often followed by profound personality changes and severe cognitive decline in which patients become wheelchair-or bed-bound, incontinent, and unable to speak or sit up.

79. A: Because of numerous side effects, glucocorticosteroids are administered orally or parentally for 5 days (prednisone, prednisolone, methylprednisolone) and then switched to inhaled steroids. If a person receives oral/parenteral glucocorticoids for longer periods, then dosages may need to be tapered. Inhaled corticosteroids include beclomethasone (Vanceril ®), budesonide (Pulmicort ®) and fluticasone propionate (Flovent ®). Corticosteroids provide anti-inflammatory action by inhibiting immune responses, decreasing edema mucus, and hyperresponsiveness.

Copyright © Mometrix Media. You have been licensed one copy of this document for personal use only. Any other reproduction or redistribution is strictly prohibited. All rights reserved.

80. C: Anticoagulation therapy is given prior to direct current cardioversion and in most cases prior to chemical cardioversion as well. There is no time to start anticoagulation when emergency defibrillation is needed. With fibrillation, blood clots may form within the heart, and when the pulse rate converts to normal, these clots can travel, increasing risk of heart attack or stroke, so the patient is usually maintained on anticoagulation (commonly warfarin) for up to 6 months after cardioversion.

81. A: Atrial septal defect is characterized by shunting of blood returning from the lungs through the left atrium back to the right atrium, and pulmonary circulation. Ventricular septal defect is characterized by left to right shunt and with Eisenmenger's syndrome (in 10%) causing increased pulmonary hypertension and right-sided heart failure. Pulmonic stenosis causes right ventricular hypertrophy from increased pressure in right ventricle and decreased pulmonary blood flow. Aortic stenosis causes left ventricular wall hypertrophy as pressure increases to overcome valvular resistance.

82. A: The fifth cranial nerve (trigeminal) is tested by lightly stroking the forehead, cheek, and jaw and having the patient open the mouth. The muscles of the jaw should be palpated for size and strength. The third cranial nerve (oculomotor) is checked with a penlight while the fourth cranial nerve (trochlear), which examines eye muscles (upward movement), is checked by having the eyes follow a moving finger vertically. The eighth cranial nerve (vestibulocochlear) is assessed for balance and hearing.

83. B: The best method to evaluate a patient's educational outcomes related to being taught a procedure is to ask the patient to do a demonstration. Patient feedback isn't a reliable indicator of ability to perform. Tests, whether oral or written, can identify what a patient knows and may be appropriate for testing general knowledge about a subject (such as diet), but knowing and doing are different skills, so demonstration is critical and allows the nurse

to provide feedback or additional training if needed.

84. C: Vacuum pressure for suctioning a tracheostomy tube is 80 to 100 mm Hg. The suction catheter should be 50% the size of the tracheostomy tube in order to allow ventilation during suctioning, and the catheter should be only inserted ≤ 0.5 cm beyond the tube to avoid damage to tissues or perforation. The catheter should be inserted without suction and intermittent suction used on withdrawal. The patient must have continuous monitoring of vital signs and respiratory status to ensure patency of tracheostomy.

85. B: Heparin-induced thrombocytopenia can cause a thrombosis syndrome that puts the patient at increased risk of thrombosis and vessel occlusion rather than hemorrhage. Because the drop in platelet count is to below 50,000 $mm^3$, this indicates this is type II (rather than transient type I), an auto immune reaction to heparin, which causes heparin-antibody complexes to form and release platelet factor 4, which in turn attracts heparin molecules and adheres to platelets and endothelial lining, stimulating thrombin and platelet clumping. Discontinuation of the heparin and treatment with direct thrombin inhibitors (Lepirudin, Argatroban®) is indicated.

86. C: This is class III. Hypovolemic shock occurs with inadequate intravascular fluid. The loss may be absolute, caused by internal shifting of fluid or external loss of fluid. Loss may also be relative, related to vasodilation, increased capillary membrane permeability from sepsis or injuries, and decreased colloidal osmotic pressure. Hypovolemic classifications include:

- Class I: <750 mL or ≤15% of total circulating volume (TCV). HR <100, BP normal.
- Class II: 750-1000 mL or 15%-20% of TCV. HR >100, BP normal.
- Class III: 1500-2000 mL or 30%-40% of TC. HR >120, BP decreased.
- Class IV: >2000 mL or >40% of TCV. HR >140, BP decreased.

Copyright © Mometrix Media. You have been licensed one copy of this document for personal use only. Any other reproduction or redistribution is strictly prohibited. All rights reserved.

87. C: A 1.5-L reservoir bag is attached and connects to the oxygen source. The bag is inflated to about 1 liter at the rate of 8 to 15 L/min before the mask is applied as the patient breathes from this reservoir. A one-way valve is part of the mask and prevents most exhaled air from being rebreathed. The non–rebreather mask can be used to deliver higher concentrations (60%-90%) of oxygen. The mask fits over the nose and mouth and is secured by an elastic strap.

88. A: The jugular venous pulse, observing the right internal jugular vein, can be used to assess right atrial function. The "a" wave that occurs with the atrial contraction can be observed in the internal jugular vein preceding the carotid pulsation. The "v" wave, after the carotid pulsation, occurs with atrial filling. The "a" wave is absent in atrial fibrillation. Large "a" waves indicate obstructed atrial blood flow. Very large (cannon) "a" waves may indicate closed tricuspid valve, AV block, junctional bradycardia,SVT, and VT. Large "v" waves occur with incompetent tricuspid valve.

89. A: Midazolam (Versed ®) is a short-acting water-soluble sedative with onset of 1 to 5 minutes, peaking in 30 minutes, and duration of about an hour (although it may last up to 6 hours). Fentanyl is a short-acting opioid with immediate onset, peaking in 10 to 15 minutes and with duration of about 20 to 45 minutes. The fentanyl/midazolam combination provides both sedation and pain control. In most cases, conscious sedation requires 6 hours of fasting prior to administration.

90. B: Popular press, including both print and other media (television, Internet) is not a valid source of information. Juried medical journals and professional physician's associations are valid because they present information based on research and best practices. Physicians on staff may also provide valid information, but should not be relied on solely as they may have bias.

91. D: V4 is placed at the left midclavicular line. The standard 12-lead ECG gives a picture of electrical activity from 12 perspectives through placement of 10 body leads. Four limb leads are placed distally on the wrists and ankles (but may be placed more proximally if necessary). Precordial leads:

- V1 right sternal border at 4th intercostal space
- V2 left sternal border at 4th intercostal space
- V3: midway between V2 and V4
- V4 left midclavicular line at 5th intercostal space
- V5 horizontal to V4 at left anterior axillary line
- V6 horizontal to V5 at left midaxillary line

92. B: A U-wave more than 1 mm high after the T-wave, AV block, and flat or inverted T-waves, are characteristic of hypokalemia. Tall, peaked T-waves with widening and increased amplitude of QRS and prolongation of the QT interval are characteristic of hyperkalemia. Dysrhythmias with prolonged PR and QT intervals and broad, flat T-waves are characteristic of hypomagnesemia. Other electrolyte imbalances are not reflected by specific ECG changes although hypermagnesemia can lead to cardiac arrest and hypercalcemia can cause dysrhythmias (similar to those of digitalis toxicity).

93. D: Hypertensive crisis is marked elevation of blood pressure that can cause severe organ damage if left untreated. It may be related to either primary or secondary hypertension, dissection of aortic aneurysm, pulmonary edema, CNS disorders, eclampsia, and failure to take medications correctly. Hypertension emergency (>120 mm Hs diastolic) requires immediate treatment to prevent organ damage. Hypertensive urgency requires treatment within a few hours, but organs are not in immediate danger. BP is lowered more slowly to avoid hypotension and organ ischemia (1/2 reduction in 6 hours, 1/3 reduction in the next 24 hours, and 1/3 reduction over 2 to 4 days).

*Copyright © Mometrix Media. You have been licensed one copy of this document for personal use only. Any other reproduction or redistribution is strictly prohibited. All rights reserved.*

94. A: Diltiazem (Cardizem ®) is a calcium channel blocker that primarily dilates coronary arteries. Capoten (Captopril ®) is an ACE inhibitor that primarily causes peripheral vasodilation and is used to decrease afterload and preload for heart failure. Nitroglycerine, a smooth muscle relaxant, primarily dilates veins and reduces preload for heart failure, unstable angina, and acute MI. Sodium nitroprusside (Nipride ®), another smooth muscle relaxant, dilates both arteries and veins, treats hypertension, and reduces afterload for heart failure.

95. D: As an advocate for the patient, the nurse must prevent possible injury to a patient: "The catheter was contaminated when it fell," states the problem. "Would you like me to get another setup or stay with the patient?" suggests a solution without assigning blame. A contaminated catheter could cause a serious infection. Reporting the team leader's behavior to the supervisor, while appropriate, does not protect the patient. Saying nothing protects only the first nurse from possible repercussions and is unprofessional conduct.

96. B: Uremic syndrome (US) related to ESRD includes erythrocytopenia because the kidney is unable to produce adequate erythropoietin in the peritubular cells, resulting in anemia. Other indications of US include thrombocytopenia leading to bleeding disorders, metabolic acidosis, as the tubular cells are unable to regulate acid-base metabolism and phosphate, sulfuric, hippuric, and lactic acids increase, leading to CHF, and weakness. Hyperkalemia occurs because the nephrons cannot excrete adequate amounts of potassium.

97. A: Increased hematocrit is a common finding with obstructive sleep apnea. OSA results from passive collapse of the pharynx during sleep, often associated with narrow or restricted upper airway (micrognathia, obesity, enlarged tonsils). It is most common in middle-age overweight males, and is exacerbated by drinking and ingesting alcohol or sedative drugs before sleeping. Symptoms include daytime somnolence, headache, cognitive impairment, depression, personality changes, recent increase in weight, and impotence. Patients often snore loudly with cycles of breath cessation caused by apneic periods of up to 60 seconds, occurring at least 30 times a night.

98. D: All staff members are responsible for identifying quality performance improvement projects. Performance improvement must be a continuous process. Continuous Quality Improvement (CQI) is a management philosophy that emphasizes the organization and the systems and processes within that organization rather than individuals. Total Quality Management (TQM) is a management philosophy that espouses a commitment to meeting the needs of the customers (patients, staff) at all levels within an organization. Both management philosophies recognize that change can be made in small steps and should involve staff at all levels.

99. B: A sodium level of 128 mEq/L indicates hyponatremia. Normal values range from 135 to 145 mEq/L. Both hypernatremia and hyponatremia can occur after cardiac surgery although hyponatremia is more common. Hyponatremia may result from loss of sodium or increase in fluid. Symptoms include:
- Irritability to lethargy to lethargy and alterations in consciousness
- Cerebral edema with seizures and coma
- Dyspnea to respiratory failure

100. D: In third-degree AV block, there are more P-waves than QRS with no clear relationship between them and an atrial rate 2-3 times the pulse rate, with an irregular PR interval. If the SA node malfunctions, the AV node fires at a lower rate, and if the AV node malfunctions, the pacemaker site in the ventricles takes over at a bradycardic rate: thus, with complete AV block, the heart still contracts but often ineffectually. The atrial P (sinus rhythm or atrial fibrillation) and the ventricular QRS (ventricular escape rhythm) are stimulated by different impulses, so

*Copyright © Mometrix Media. You have been licensed one copy of this document for personal use only. Any other reproduction or redistribution is strictly prohibited. All rights reserved.*

there is AV dissociation. The heart can't compensate with exertion.

101. B: Advocacy is working for the best interests of the patient, despite personal values in conflict and assisting patients to have access to appropriate resources. Moral agency is the ability to recognize needs and take action to influence the outcome of a conflict or decision. Agency is openness and recognition of issues and a willingness to act. Collaboration is working together to achieve better results.

102 C: Subarachnoid hemorrhage usually presents initially with severe headache, nausea and vomiting, nuchal rigidity, palsy related to cranial nerve compression, retinal hemorrhages, and papilledema. Late complications include hyponatremia and hydrocephalus. Symptoms worsen as intracranial pressure rises, progressing to confusion and drowsiness, stupor, coma, and decerebrate rigidity. SAH may occur after trauma but is common from rupture of berry aneurysm or an arteriovenous malformation (AVM). SAH may also be caused by neoplasms, sickle cell disease, infection, hemophilia, and leukemia.

103. C: The AICD, used to control tachycardia and fibrillation, provides on-demand (synchronous) small electrical impulses to the atrial or ventricular myocardium to slow the heart when the pulse rate increases to a preset rate. If fibrillation occurs, a higher energy shock is delivered. It takes 5 to 15 seconds for the device to detect abnormalities in the pulse rate and more than one shock may be required, so fainting may occur. Some devices can function as both a pacemaker and an ICD for those with episodes of both bradycardia and tachycardia.

104. B: Urinary output should be maintained at >25 mL/hr consistent with fluid intake. Output should be measured every half hour for the first 4 hours and then every 8 hours if output is normal. Specific gravity is monitored to determine the kidneys' ability to concentrate urine, and the serum creatinine and electrolytes indicate the kidneys' ability to excrete waste products. Renal damage can occur from inadequate perfusion, hemolysis, decreased cardiac output, and the use of vasopressor medications to control blood pressure.

105. D: Symptoms typical of a dissecting descending aortic aneurysm include severe, intense knife-life posterior pain between the scapulas, nausea, and vomiting. Patients may be cold and clammy. Dissection of the ascending thoracic aorta results in similar symptoms, but the pain is in the anterior chest. Pain with dissection does not generally increase in intensity, as it is severe at onset when tearing occurs. Peripheral arteries may be involved, and this can cause numbness, tingling, and evidence of vascular insufficiency in an affected limb.

106. C: The nurse should face the patient at a distance of 2 to 6 feet, use a normal tone of voice and short sentences, utilize gestures, and provide assistive devices as necessary, including writing materials and TDD phone/relay service. Many hearing-impaired patients use some degree of lip-reading, so the nurse should not chew, or eat while speaking to the patient. If patients are deaf and know sign language, interpreters should be used for important communication, and the nurse should face the patient during communication, not the interpreter.

107. C: The best determinant of teaching effectiveness is behavior modification noted through observation and measurement. Many times compliance rates are based on patient reports, but these are not always accurate. Satisfaction does not necessarily lead to compliance. A knowledgeable instructor is important, but knowledge does not always relate to teaching abilities.

108. B: Brownish discoloration (hemosiderin) around ankles and anterior tibial areas is a sign of peripheral venous insufficiency. Other signs include varicosities, venous dermatitis, irregular ulcers on medial or lateral malleolus or anterior tibial area and moderate to severe edema. Peripheral pulses are often weak or absent with

Copyright © Mometrix Media. You have been licensed one copy of this document for personal use only. Any other reproduction or redistribution is strictly prohibited. All rights reserved.

arterial insufficiency, and pain is either intermittent or constant and severe. With venous insufficiency, pulses are present, and pain is aching and cramping.

109. B: While the international normalized ratio (INR) is individualized depending on baseline readings, a normal INR is approximately 1. Those receiving warfarin for atrial fibrillation are maintained at an INR of 2 to 3. The INR for prophylaxis for deep vein thrombosis is 1.5 to 2 and for pulmonary emboli and mechanical heart values is 3 to 4. The higher the number, the greater the anticoagulation effect, therefore a level greater than 4 may put the patient at risk for hemorrhage.

110. C: According to Knowles, adult learners tend to be practical and goal-oriented, so they like to remain organized and keep the goal in mind while learning. Other characteristics include:

- Self-direction: Adults like active involvement and responsibility.
- Knowledgeable: Adults can relate new material to information with which they are familiar by life experience or education.
- Relevancy orientation: Adults like to know how they will use information.
- Motivated: Adults like to see evidence of their achievement, for example, through the receipt of a certificate.

111. A: Contraindications to thrombolytic therapy include aortic aneurysm, hemorrhagic stroke, recent surgery, or bleeding. While ideally, thrombolytic therapy should be administered within 90 minutes of onset of symptoms, it may be given within 6 hours for tenecteplase and within 12 hours for other thrombolytics. History of any type of stroke within 2 months or AVM precludes thrombolytic therapy. Severe hypertension (>210/130 mm Hg) that is uncontrolled by medications or that occurs with retinal-vascular disease is also a contraindication.

112. B: Cardiogenic shock is characterized by hypotension with systolic BP <90 mm Hg, tachycardia >100 bpm with weak, thready pulse, and dysrhythmias, decreased heart sounds, chest pain, tachypnea and basilar râles, pallor, and cool moist skin. Cardiogenic shock is often secondary to MI that reduces the contractibility of the ventricles and interferes with the pumping mechanism of the heart decreasing oxygen perfusion. Characteristics include increased preload and afterload and decreased contractibility, resulting in decreased cardiac output and increased systemic vascular resistance causing pulmonary edema and right ventricular failure.

113. B: Dobutamine is used to treat low cardiac output after cardiac surgery. Nitroprusside decreases blood pressure and afterload. Dopamine treats shock and hypotension for patients who required volume resuscitation. Isoproterenol is used to stimulate the heart in patients with severe bradycardia. Other drugs include nitroglycerine, used to prevent spasm in arterial grafts and to reduce preload and afterload, and epinephrine is used to treat low cardiac output related to shock. Milrinone is also used to low cardiac output. Phenylephrine, norepinephrine, and vasopressin increase systemic vascular resistance and blood pressure, and are used to treat shock.

114. A: The patient with acute heart failure will most likely receive a diuretic to reduce fluid and sodium retention, a vasodilator to reduce blood pressure, digoxin to increase contractibility of the weakened ventricles, and an anticoagulant because of the enlarged ventricles and atrial fibrillation, which increase the risk of thromboembolia. Other treatments include weight monitoring, low sodium diet, and activity restriction.

115. B: Sinus tachycardia is characterized by pulse >100 bpm. The rapid pulse decreases diastolic filling time and reduces cardiac output with resultant hypotension and pulmonary edema. Bradycardia is characterized by pulse <60 bpm. Sinus is common in children and young

Copyright © Mometrix Media. You have been licensed one copy of this document for personal use only. Any other reproduction or redistribution is strictly prohibited. All rights reserved.

adults, but may occur with vagal stimulation from suctioning, vomiting, or defecating. Premature atrial contractions are essentially extra beats caused by an electrical impulse to the atrium before the sinus node impulse, resulting in an irregular pulse.

116. D: AIDS is diagnosed with HIV infection, CD4 count <200 cells/mm³, and AIDS-defining condition, such as opportunistic infections (cytomegalovirus, tuberculosis), wasting syndrome, neoplasms (Kaposi's sarcoma) or AIDS dementia complex. Patients with AIDS may present with many types of symptoms, depending on the AIDS-defining condition, but more than half exhibit fever, lymphadenopathy, pharyngitis, rash, and myalgia/arthralgia.

117. D: These symptoms, including the abnormal heart sound (ejection click), are common to aortic valve stenosis. The aortic valve controlling the flow of blood from the left ventricle narrows, causing the left ventricular wall to thicken. Aortic stenosis may result from a birth defect or from damage caused by childhood rheumatic fever. Coronary artery disease is not directly associated with abnormal heart sounds although gallop rhythms can occur with related ventricular hypertrophy. Mitral valve stenosis may cause an opening snap, while pericarditis causes a friction rub.

118. D: Atrial arrhythmias, including fibrillation, flutter, and tachycardia, are very common after cardiac surgery, occurring in more than half of patients with valvular surgery. Arrhythmias occur usually in the first 2-3 postoperative days and are often transient but may recur. Arrhythmias are often related to surgical manipulation. Treatment includes digoxin, β-blockers, calcium channel blockers, and amiodarone (often given preoperatively for 7 days to reduce incidence of postoperative arrhythmias. Electrical cardioversion may be indicated after 24 hours if sinus rhythm remains abnormal.

119. A: A short-acting intravenous loop diuretic, such as furosemide (Lasix ®) or bumetanide

(Bumex ®) is indicated to rapidly reduce fluid retention and decrease pulmonary edema. Spironolactone and eplerenone are potassium-spring diuretics that have weaker diuretic actions than loop diuretics. Hydrochlorothiazide is a long-acting thiazide diuretic given as a first line treatment for hypertension rather than for acute crises.

120. C: SIRS symptoms may include leukocytosis or leukopenia. SIRS is diagnosed with 2 of the following symptoms:

- Leukocytosis (>12,000 mm³) or leukopenia (<4000 mm³).
- Elevated (>38°C) or subnormal rectal temperature (<36°C).
- Tachypnea or $PaCO_2$ <32 mm Hg.
- Tachycardia.

SIRS, a generalized inflammatory response affecting many organ systems, may be caused by infectious or noninfectious agents, such as trauma, burns, adrenal insufficiency, pulmonary embolism, and drug overdose. If an infectious agent (such as Streptococcus pneumonia or Staphylococcus aureus) is identified or suspected, SIRS may be an aspect of sepsis.

121. A: With type I HITTS, heparin is continued while monitoring platelet count. This condition is transient but typically resolves without intervention. Type II is an autoimmune reaction to heparin that occurs in 3% to 5% of those receiving unfractionated heparin and also occurs with low-molecular weight heparin. It is characterized by low platelets (<50,000 mm³) that are ≥50% below baseline. Onset is 5 to14 days but can occur within hours of reheparinization. Heparin-antibody complexes form and release platelet factor 4 (PF4), which attracts heparin molecules and adheres to platelets and endothelial lining; stimulating thrombin and platelet clumping.

Copyright © Mometrix Media. You have been licensed one copy of this document for personal use only. Any other reproduction or redistribution is strictly prohibited. All rights reserved.

122. A: The translator should have training in medical vocabulary for both languages because just speaking the languages well does not mean that the translator will adequately translate specialized vocabulary. It is not necessary for the translator to know the patient's history as the translator's job is only to translate what is said, not add to it or interpret it based on prior knowledge. While on-site translators are ideal, translation can be done with a speakerphone at a distance.

123. A: A dissecting 6-cm aneurysm in the ascending aorta is a medical emergency and requires immediate repair. Abdominal aneurysm (saccular or fusiform) repair is often delayed until it reaches >5.5 cm unless an aneurysm is rapidly expanding in size. Thoracic aneurysm repair is also typically delayed until the aneurysm reaches >5.5 cm, but those with Marfan's syndrome may be advised to have surgery at 5 cm due to increased risk.

124. C: If a patient is having a generalized (grand mal) seizure, the nurse should try to position the patient on one side with the head flexed forward to allow the tongue to fall forward so that it doesn't obstruct the airway to prevent aspiration of saliva and mucus. Padding should be placed under the head to prevent injury from contact with a hard surface. The patient should not be restrained as this can cause injury. Clothing should be loosened and furniture moved out of the way. If the patient is in bed, the pillow should be removed and side rails raised.

125. D: ACE inhibitors are contraindicated with renal failure, as one of the most serious side effects is renal impairment, especially in patients also taking diuretics and NSAIDs. ACE inhibitors are commonly used to treat hypertension and heart failure. They are often combined with diuretics, such as thiazide for hypertension or Lasix ® for heart failure. ACE inhibitors are sometimes given to those with diabetes mellitus to prevent diabetic neuropathy.

Copyright © Mometrix Media. You have been licensed one copy of this document for personal use only. Any other reproduction or redistribution is strictly prohibited. All rights reserved.

# Secret Key #1 - Time is Your Greatest Enemy

## Pace Yourself

Wear a watch. At the beginning of the test, check the time (or start a chronometer on your watch to count the minutes), and check the time after every few questions to make sure you are "on schedule."

If you are forced to speed up, do it efficiently. Usually one or more answer choices can be eliminated without too much difficulty. Above all, don't panic. Don't speed up and just begin guessing at random choices. By pacing yourself, and continually monitoring your progress against your watch, you will always know exactly how far ahead or behind you are with your available time. If you find that you are one minute behind on the test, don't skip one question without spending any time on it, just to catch back up. Take 15 fewer seconds on the next four questions, and after four questions you'll have caught back up. Once you catch back up, you can continue working each problem at your normal pace.

Furthermore, don't dwell on the problems that you were rushed on. If a problem was taking up too much time and you made a hurried guess, it must be difficult. The difficult questions are the ones you are most likely to miss anyway, so it isn't a big loss. It is better to end with more time than you need than to run out of time.

Lastly, sometimes it is beneficial to slow down if you are constantly getting ahead of time. You are always more likely to catch a careless mistake by working more slowly than quickly, and among very high-scoring test takers (those who are likely to have lots of time left over), careless errors affect the score more than mastery of material.

# Secret Key #2 - Guessing is not Guesswork

You probably know that guessing is a good idea - unlike other standardized tests, there is no penalty for getting a wrong answer. Even if you have no idea about a question, you still have a 20-25% chance of getting it right.

Most test takers do not understand the impact that proper guessing can have on their score. Unless you score extremely high, guessing will significantly contribute to your final score.

## Monkeys Take the Test

What most test takers don't realize is that to insure that 20-25% chance, you have to guess randomly. If you put 20 monkeys in a room to take this test, assuming they answered once per question and behaved themselves, on average they would get 20-25% of the questions correct. Put 20 test takers in the room, and the average will be much lower among guessed questions. Why?

1. The test writers intentionally writes deceptive answer choices that "look" right. A test taker has no idea about a question, so picks the "best looking" answer, which is often wrong. The monkey has no idea what looks good and what doesn't, so will consistently be lucky about 20-25% of the time.
2. Test takers will eliminate answer choices from the guessing pool based on a hunch or intuition. Simple but correct answers often get excluded, leaving a 0% chance of being correct. The monkey has no clue, and often gets lucky with the best choice.

This is why the process of elimination endorsed by most test courses is flawed and detrimental to your performance- test takers don't guess, they make an ignorant stab in the dark that is usually worse than random.

Copyright © Mometrix Media. You have been licensed one copy of this document for personal use only. Any other reproduction or redistribution is strictly prohibited. All rights reserved.

## $5 Challenge

Let me introduce one of the most valuable ideas of this course- the $5 challenge:

*You only mark your "best guess" if you are willing to bet $5 on it.*
*You only eliminate choices from guessing if you are willing to bet $5 on it.*

Why $5? Five dollars is an amount of money that is small yet not insignificant, and can really add up fast (20 questions could cost you $100). Likewise, each answer choice on one question of the test will have a small impact on your overall score, but it can really add up to a lot of points in the end.

The process of elimination IS valuable. The following shows your chance of guessing it right:

| If you eliminate wrong answer choices until only this many remain: | 1 | 2 | 3 |
|---|---|---|---|
| Chance of getting it correct: | 100% | 50% | 33% |

However, if you accidentally eliminate the right answer or go on a hunch for an incorrect answer, your chances drop dramatically: to 0%. By guessing among all the answer choices, you are GUARANTEED to have a shot at the right answer.

That's why the $5 test is so valuable- if you give up the advantage and safety of a pure guess, it had better be worth the risk.

What we still haven't covered is how to be sure that whatever guess you make is truly random. Here's the easiest way:

*Always pick the first answer choice among those remaining.*

Such a technique means that you have decided, **before you see a single test question**, exactly how you are going to guess- and since the order of choices tells you nothing about which one is correct, this guessing technique is perfectly random.

This section is not meant to scare you away from making educated guesses or eliminating choices- you just need to define when a choice is worth eliminating. The $5 test, along with a pre-defined random guessing strategy, is the best way to make sure you reap all of the benefits of guessing.

# Secret Key #3 - Practice Smarter, Not Harder

Many test takers delay the test preparation process because they dread the awful amounts of practice time they think necessary to succeed on the test. We have refined an effective method that will take you only a fraction of the time.

There are a number of "obstacles" in your way to succeed. Among these are answering questions, finishing in time, and mastering test-taking strategies. All must be executed on the day of the test at peak performance, or your score will suffer. The test is a mental marathon that has a large impact on your future.

Just like a marathon runner, it is important to work your way up to the full challenge. So first you just worry about questions, and then time, and finally strategy:

## Success Strategy

1. Find a good source for practice tests.
2. If you are willing to make a larger time investment, consider using more than one study guide- often the different approaches of multiple authors will help you "get" difficult concepts.
3. Take a practice test with no time constraints, with all study helps "open book." Take your time with questions and focus on applying strategies.
4. Take a practice test with time constraints, with all guides "open book."
5. Take a final practice test with no open material and time limits

*Copyright © Mometrix Media. You have been licensed one copy of this document for personal use only. Any other reproduction or redistribution is strictly prohibited. All rights reserved.*

If you have time to take more practice tests, just repeat step 5. By gradually exposing yourself to the full rigors of the test environment, you will condition your mind to the stress of test day and maximize your success.

# Secret Key #4 - Prepare, Don't Procrastinate

Let me state an obvious fact: if you take the test three times, you will get three different scores. This is due to the way you feel on test day, the level of preparedness you have, and, despite the test writers' claims to the contrary, some tests WILL be easier for you than others.

Since your future depends so much on your score, you should maximize your chances of success. In order to maximize the likelihood of success, you've got to prepare in advance. This means taking practice tests and spending time learning the information and test taking strategies you will need to succeed.

Never take the test as a "practice" test, expecting that you can just take it again if you need to. Feel free to take sample tests on your own, but when you go to take the official test, be prepared, be focused, and do your best the first time!

# Secret Key #5 - Test Yourself

Everyone knows that time is money. There is no need to spend too much of your time or too little of your time preparing for the test. You should only spend as much of your precious time preparing as is necessary for you to get the score you need.

Once you have taken a practice test under real conditions of time constraints, then you will know if you are ready for the test or not.

If you have scored extremely high the first time that you take the practice test, then there is not much point in spending countless hours studying. You are already there.

Benchmark your abilities by retaking practice tests and seeing how much you have improved. Once you score high enough to guarantee success, then you are ready.

If you have scored well below where you need, then knuckle down and begin studying in earnest. Check your improvement regularly through the use of practice tests under real conditions. Above all, don't worry, panic, or give up. The key is perseverance!

Then, when you go to take the test, remain confident and remember how well you did on the practice tests. If you can score high enough on a practice test, then you can do the same on the real thing.

# General Strategies

The most important thing you can do is to ignore your fears and jump into the test immediately- do not be overwhelmed by any strange-sounding terms. You have to jump into the test like jumping into a pool- all at once is the easiest way.

## Make Predictions

As you read and understand the question, try to guess what the answer will be. Remember that several of the answer choices are wrong, and once you begin reading them, your mind will immediately become cluttered with answer choices designed to throw you off. Your mind is typically the most focused immediately after you have read the question and digested its contents. If you can, try to predict what the correct answer will be. You may be surprised at what you can predict.

Quickly scan the choices and see if your prediction is in the listed answer choices. If it is, then you can be quite confident that you have

Copyright © Mometrix Media. You have been licensed one copy of this document for personal use only. Any other reproduction or redistribution is strictly prohibited. All rights reserved.

the right answer. It still won't hurt to check the other answer choices, but most of the time, you've got it!

## Answer the Question

It may seem obvious to only pick answer choices that answer the question, but the test writers can create some excellent answer choices that are wrong. Don't pick an answer just because it sounds right, or you believe it to be true. It MUST answer the question. Once you've made your selection, always go back and check it against the question and make sure that you didn't misread the question, and the answer choice does answer the question posed.

## Benchmark

After you read the first answer choice, decide if you think it sounds correct or not. If it doesn't, move on to the next answer choice. If it does, mentally mark that answer choice. This doesn't mean that you've definitely selected it as your answer choice, it just means that it's the best you've seen thus far. Go ahead and read the next choice. If the next choice is worse than the one you've already selected, keep going to the next answer choice. If the next choice is better than the choice you've already selected, mentally mark the new answer choice as your best guess.

The first answer choice that you select becomes your standard. Every other answer choice must be benchmarked against that standard. That choice is correct until proven otherwise by another answer choice beating it out. Once you've decided that no other answer choice seems as good, do one final check to ensure that your answer choice answers the question posed.

## Valid Information

Don't discount any of the information provided in the question. Every piece of information may be necessary to determine the correct answer. None of the information in the question is there to throw you off (while the answer choices will certainly have information to throw you off). If two seemingly unrelated topics are discussed, don't ignore either. You can be confident there is

a relationship, or it wouldn't be included in the question, and you are probably going to have to determine what is that relationship to find the answer.

## Avoid "Fact Traps"

Don't get distracted by a choice that is factually true. Your search is for the answer that answers the question. Stay focused and don't fall for an answer that is true but incorrect. Always go back to the question and make sure you're choosing an answer that actually answers the question and is not just a true statement. An answer can be factually correct, but it MUST answer the question asked. Additionally, two answers can both be seemingly correct, so be sure to read all of the answer choices, and make sure that you get the one that BEST answers the question.

## Milk the Question

Some of the questions may throw you completely off. They might deal with a subject you have not been exposed to, or one that you haven't reviewed in years. While your lack of knowledge about the subject will be a hindrance, the question itself can give you many clues that will help you find the correct answer. Read the question carefully and look for clues. Watch particularly for adjectives and nouns describing difficult terms or words that you don't recognize. Regardless of if you completely understand a word or not, replacing it with a synonym either provided or one you more familiar with may help you to understand what the questions are asking. Rather than wracking your mind about specific detailed information concerning a difficult term or word, try to use mental substitutes that are easier to understand.

## The Trap of Familiarity

Don't just choose a word because you recognize it. On difficult questions, you may not recognize a number of words in the answer choices. The test writers don't put "make-believe" words on the test; so don't think that just because you only recognize all the words in one answer choice means that answer choice must be correct. If you only recognize words in one answer choice,

*Copyright © Mometrix Media. You have been licensed one copy of this document for personal use only. Any other reproduction or redistribution is strictly prohibited. All rights reserved.*

then focus on that one. Is it correct? Try your best to determine if it is correct. If it is, that is great, but if it doesn't, eliminate it. Each word and answer choice you eliminate increases your chances of getting the question correct, even if you then have to guess among the unfamiliar choices.

## Eliminate Answers

Eliminate choices as soon as you realize they are wrong. But be careful! Make sure you consider all of the possible answer choices. Just because one appears right, doesn't mean that the next one won't be even better! The test writers will usually put more than one good answer choice for every question, so read all of them. Don't worry if you are stuck between two that seem right. By getting down to just two remaining possible choices, your odds are now 50/50. Rather than wasting too much time, play the odds. You are guessing, but guessing wisely, because you've been able to knock out some of the answer choices that you know are wrong. If you are eliminating choices and realize that the last answer choice you are left with is also obviously wrong, don't panic. Start over and consider each choice again. There may easily be something that you missed the first time and will realize on the second pass.

## Tough Questions

If you are stumped on a problem or it appears too hard or too difficult, don't waste time. Move on! Remember though, if you can quickly check for obviously incorrect answer choices, your chances of guessing correctly are greatly improved. Before you completely give up, at least try to knock out a couple of possible answers. Eliminate what you can and then guess at the remaining answer choices before moving on.

## Brainstorm

If you get stuck on a difficult question, spend a few seconds quickly brainstorming. Run through the complete list of possible answer choices. Look at each choice and ask yourself, "Could this answer the question satisfactorily?"

Go through each answer choice and consider it independently of the other. By systematically going through all possibilities, you may find something that you would otherwise overlook. Remember that when you get stuck, it's important to try to keep moving.

## Read Carefully

Understand the problem. Read the question and answer choices carefully. Don't miss the question because you misread the terms. You have plenty of time to read each question thoroughly and make sure you understand what is being asked. Yet a happy medium must be attained, so don't waste too much time. You must read carefully, but efficiently.

## Face Value

When in doubt, use common sense. Always accept the situation in the problem at face value. Don't read too much into it. These problems will not require you to make huge leaps of logic. The test writers aren't trying to throw you off with a cheap trick. If you have to go beyond creativity and make a leap of logic in order to have an answer choice answer the question, then you should look at the other answer choices. Don't overcomplicate the problem by creating theoretical relationships or explanations that will warp time or space. These are normal problems rooted in reality. It's just that the applicable relationship or explanation may not be readily apparent and you have to figure things out. Use your common sense to interpret anything that isn't clear.

## Prefixes

If you're having trouble with a word in the question or answer choices, try dissecting it. Take advantage of every clue that the word might include. Prefixes and suffixes can be a huge help. Usually they allow you to determine a basic meaning. Pre- means before, post- means after, pro - is positive, de- is negative. From these prefixes and suffixes, you can get an idea of the general meaning of the word and try to put it into context. Beware though of any traps. Just because con is the opposite of pro, doesn't

Copyright © Mometrix Media. You have been licensed one copy of this document for personal use only. Any other reproduction or redistribution is strictly prohibited. All rights reserved.

necessarily mean congress is the opposite of progress!

## Hedge Phrases

Watch out for critical "hedge" phrases, such as likely, may, can, will often, sometimes, often, almost, mostly, usually, generally, rarely, sometimes. Question writers insert these hedge phrases to cover every possibility. Often an answer choice will be wrong simply because it leaves no room for exception. Avoid answer choices that have definitive words like "exactly," and "always".

## Switchback Words

Stay alert for "switchbacks". These are the words and phrases frequently used to alert you to shifts in thought. The most common switchback word is "but". Others include although, however, nevertheless, on the other hand, even though, while, in spite of, despite, regardless of.

## New Information

Correct answer choices will rarely have completely new information included. Answer choices typically are straightforward reflections of the material asked about and will directly relate to the question. If a new piece of information is included in an answer choice that doesn't even seem to relate to the topic being asked about, then that answer choice is likely incorrect. All of the information needed to answer the question is usually provided for you, and so you should not have to make guesses that are unsupported or choose answer choices that require unknown information that cannot be reasoned on its own.

## Time Management

On technical questions, don't get lost on the technical terms. Don't spend too much time on any one question. If you don't know what a term means, then since you don't have a dictionary, odds are you aren't going to get much further. You should immediately recognize terms as whether or not you know them. If you don't,

work with the other clues that you have, the other answer choices and terms provided, but don't waste too much time trying to figure out a difficult term.

## Contextual Clues

Look for contextual clues. An answer can be right but not correct. The contextual clues will help you find the answer that is most right and is correct. Understand the context in which a phrase or statement is made. This will help you make important distinctions.

## Don't Panic

Panicking will not answer any questions for you. Therefore, it isn't helpful. When you first see the question, if your mind goes blank, take a deep breath. Force yourself to mechanically go through the steps of solving the problem and using the strategies you've learned.

## Pace Yourself

Don't get clock fever. It's easy to be overwhelmed when you're looking at a page full of questions, your mind is full of random thoughts and feeling confused, and the clock is ticking down faster than you would like. Calm down and maintain the pace that you have set for yourself. As long as you are on track by monitoring your pace, you are guaranteed to have enough time for yourself. When you get to the last few minutes of the test, it may seem like you won't have enough time left, but if you only have as many questions as you should have left at that point, then you're right on track!

## Answer Selection

The best way to pick an answer choice is to eliminate all of those that are wrong, until only one is left and confirm that is the correct answer. Sometimes though, an answer choice may immediately look right. Be careful! Take a second to make sure that the other choices are not equally obvious. Don't make a hasty mistake. There are only two times that you should stop before checking other answers. First is when you are positive that the answer choice you have

*Copyright © Mometrix Media. You have been licensed one copy of this document for personal use only. Any other reproduction or redistribution is strictly prohibited. All rights reserved.*

selected is correct. Second is when time is almost out and you have to make a quick guess!

## Check Your Work

Since you will probably not know every term listed and the answer to every question, it is important that you get credit for the ones that you do know. Don't miss any questions through careless mistakes. If at all possible, try to take a second to look back over your answer selection and make sure you've selected the correct answer choice and haven't made a costly careless mistake (such as marking an answer choice that you didn't mean to mark). This quick double check should more than pay for itself in caught mistakes for the time it costs.

## Beware of Directly Quoted Answers

Sometimes an answer choice will repeat word for word a portion of the question or reference section. However, beware of such exact duplication – it may be a trap! More than likely, the correct choice will paraphrase or summarize a point, rather than being exactly the same wording.

## Slang

Scientific sounding answers are better than slang ones. An answer choice that begins "To compare the outcomes…" is much more likely to be correct than one that begins "Because some people insisted…"

## Extreme Statements

Avoid wild answers that throw out highly controversial ideas that are proclaimed as established fact. An answer choice that states the "process should be used in certain situations, if…" is much more likely to be correct than one that states the "process should be discontinued completely." The first is a calm rational statement and doesn't even make a definitive, uncompromising stance, using a hedge word "if" to provide wiggle room, whereas the second choice is a radical idea and far more extreme.

## Answer Choice Families

When you have two or more answer choices that are direct opposites or parallels, one of them is usually the correct answer. For instance, if one answer choice states "x increases" and another answer choice states "x decreases" or "y increases," then those two or three answer choices are very similar in construction and fall into the same family of answer choices. A family of answer choices is when two or three answer choices are very similar in construction, and yet often have a directly opposite meaning. Usually the correct answer choice will be in that family of answer choices. The "odd man out" or answer choice that doesn't seem to fit the parallel construction of the other answer choices is more likely to be incorrect.

*Copyright © Mometrix Media. You have been licensed one copy of this document for personal use only. Any other reproduction or redistribution is strictly prohibited. All rights reserved.*